FABULOUS FACE

BHARTI VYAS

with Jane Warren

Thorsons

By the same author:

Simply Ayurveda: Discover your type to transform your life (with Jane Warren)
Simply Radiant (with Jane Warren)
Beauty Wisdom: The secret of looking and feeling great (with Claire Haggard)

Thorsons
An Imprint of HarperCollins*Publishers*
77–85 Fulham Palace Road,
Hammersmith, London W6 8JB

The Thorsons website address is:
www.thorsons.com

Thorsons

and *Thorsons*
are trademarks of HarperCollins*Publishers* Limited

Published by Thorsons 2002

10 9 8 7 6 5 4 3 2 1

Studio photography by Dave King
Images p. vi © Simon Wilkinson/Getty Images; p. xii © Darren Robb/Getty Images; p. 22 © Nick
Clements/Getty Images; p. 64 © Johnny Hernandez/Getty Images; p. 68 © Peter Nicholson/Getty
Images; p. 79 © David Roth/Getty Images; p. 88 © Vincent Besnault/Getty Images; p. 92 © Gary
Buss/Getty Images; p. 162 © Deborah Jaffe/Getty Images; p. 166 © Jerome Tisne/Getty Images

A catalogue record for this book is
available from the British Library

ISBN 0 00 712373 6

Printed and bound in the UK by
The Bath Press

contents

Acknowledgements v

Introduction vii

Nature

- **Your Skin** • 2

  What Is the Skin? 2

  Your Skin Type 5

  Routines for All Types 9

  Feeding Your Skin from Within 18

  Signs of Ageing 19

  Facial Hair 26

  Skin Disorders and Blemishes, and

  How to Treat Them 27

  How Sunshine Affects Your Skin 37

  Home-made Cosmetics 40

- **Your Hair** • 49

  How to Frame Your Face 49

  How to Disguise Specific Features 52

  Hair Types 53

  Caring for Different Hair Conditions 53

  Hair Disorders 56

  Colouring Your Hair 59

  Home-made Hair Treatments and Treats 61

- **Your Teeth** • 69

  Teeth and Gum Health 70

  Your Tongue 72

  Natural Tooth Whiteners 72

  Mouthwashes 73

- **Your Eyes** • 77

  Tired Eyes 78

  General Eye Care 82

  Eyelashes 83

  Eyebrow Shaping 84

- **Facial Massages and Exercises** • 93

  Bharti's Clearing Head and Scalp

  Massage 94

  Acupressure Treats 101

  Facial Lymphatic Massage 103

  How to Give Yourself a Facial

  Massage 106

  Facial Exercises 113

Nurture

Make-up • 126
Make-up Secrets with Armand 127
Breakout: Clever Colour 131
Make-up for Ageing Skin 141
Armand's Guide to the Cosmetic
Jargon Jungle 143
Armand's Top Ten Professional
Insights 144
Natural Make-up Tips 146
Label-watching 153

Clinic Treatments • 156
Botox 157
Collagen Instant Therapy 157

Mayo-lift 158
Eyelash Perm 159
Fruit Acid Peels 159
Laser Hair Removal 160
Laser Skin Resurfacing 161
Micro-dermabrasion 163
Restylane 163
Semi-permanent Make-up 164
Transdermal Electrolysis (TE)
System 165

Dental Treatments • 166
How to Achieve the Hollywood
Smile 168

Resources 175
Further Reading 178
Index 180

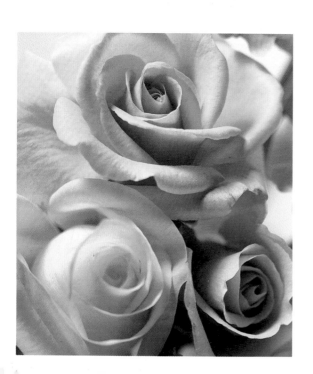

dedication

To all my clients and readers who have made my philosophy a way of life, proving that beauty wisdom is both simple and practical to put into practice.

I would like to dedicate this book also to my colleagues at Tesco who helped to make my vision come true with their Bharti Vyas Skin Wisdom beauty products. I believe that it is everybody's right to look and feel good and I aim to give them the right tools to do so.

acknowledgements

To my beloved husband, Raja; my daughters Shailu and Pritti, whose unconditional love and support have made everything possible for me; Jane Warren, a true professional and a pleasure to work with; Armand, an inspiration with make-up; Jacqueline and Patrick Grattan, sincere appreciation; all my team at Thorsons, especially my editor Wanda Whiteley, Belinda Budge, Meg Slyfield and Jo Lal; my literary agent, Caroline Shott; all the staff at my clinics, particularly Magda Reggio; my friends Lorraine Kelly at GMTV, Lorna Frame, *Daily Express* Health and Beauty Editor, Juliette Kellow at *Top Santé*, Fiona Wright and Colette Harris at *Here's Health*, Eve Cameron, Editor of *She* magazine, Ash Kamar, Michael Van Stratton, Caroline Davies at *Black Hair & Beauty*, Sameena and Sarwar Saeed at *Asian Woman* magazine; and to all the journalists and television producers who have always supported me and believed in my work.

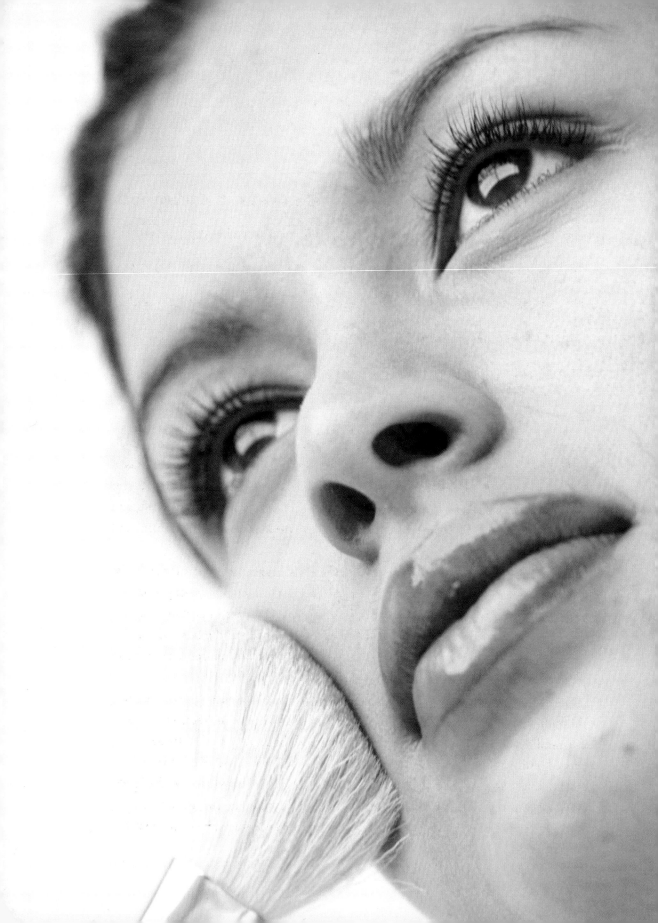

introduction

This book contains all you need to know about beauty and health treatments for your face, including your teeth, hair, scalp and eyes. It's a clear, comprehensive facial beauty bible. This is a book to browse. I am not going to insist you read it from cover to cover – instead, dip in for insights into facial care. Life is too short not to feel good about yourself, so treat yourself to an insight into ways to enhance your confidence.

The book is organized into two sections. The first, *Nature*, is a home-care section which includes techniques and approaches you can use by yourself or with your partner or a friend. In the second section, *Nurture*, I reveal the trade secrets of leading make-up artists, the more advanced clinic-based therapies for giving your face that extra lift, and dental techniques used by cosmetic dentists to achieve the ultimate in enhancement and Hollywood gloss.

As a source of confidence, our face is the most important part of our body, yet, together with our neck and ears, it is also the most vulnerable and exposed part of our anatomy. Hands are also exposed, but although they are important they are not considered the visible seat of personality in the same way as the face, which also contains crucial perceptual functions. It is true to say that the face, more than any other part of our physiology, transcends the merely mechanical.

Skin is the connection between our inner and outer worlds, and reflects what is going on in both. People look at your skin, hair and eyes in an attempt to assess your mood, understand your character, and to make judgements about your health. In our faces, burdened with all this social significance, we are truly laid bare. And all the time we are peering out, feeling powerless when our visage does not reflect how we feel on the inside.

We all know how a spot or a bad hair day can destroy our confidence. Understanding how your face works – and no two skin types are ever the same – and what you can do to correct imbalances is therefore about much more than just following a superficial beauty regimen; it is directly connected to your very image of yourself.

The face tells us a lot of things, in the same way that we can look at posture and see how tension is affecting us. When someone walks into my clinic with hunched shoulders, for example, I can tell they probably do not have enough oxygen in their blood – their lungs are simply not able to work to full capacity in that cramped ribcage, and this means that there is a good chance that the oxygen level in their body is not high enough to metabolize the nutrients in their food completely so that it releases all its potential energy. Likewise, in assessing health I look to see whether my client has firm skin, bright wide-open eyes, full lips, a defined lip-line, and an even skin tone. Instead, if I observe leathery skin, open pores or tired or droopy eyes, I will ask questions to find out more; are they feeling unwell, taking medication or drinking more than they should? Then we set out to change their life.

not just skin deep

As I always say to my clients, the state of your face is allied to your internal constitution, a reflection of the state of your inner body. Beauty on the outside really does begin on the inside, and nowhere is that more true than on the surface of the facial skin, the first area to register internal problems. If the system is not in balance, no amount of lotion is going to mask that. The most expensive skin cream will be a waste of money if you aren't looking after your stress level, your diet and the amount of exercise you are getting. Drinking lots of water to cleanse yourself from within, eating healthily to avoid a build-up of toxins, and getting plenty of sleep to allow your body and brain to repair themselves, are attitudes to beauty and well-being that must be the cornerstones of your approach.

Superficial changes are not enough. I believe that everyone has the power within themselves to transform the way they look and feel in only 12 weeks by cutting out wheat and dairy products – which can lead to flu-like symptoms, bloatedness, tiredness and headaches – drinking a glass of water every hour, and eating fresh fruit and vegetables.

When I was training to be a beauty therapist, one of my husband's friends, a herbalist in Kenya, told me that if your gut and respiratory tract are not clean, you will never have good skin. This is why cutting down on your wheat intake can help your skin look better. Wheat contains gluten, which lines the intestines and delays the absorption of nutrients in the digestive tract. Cutting down on your dairy intake helps give the respiratory tract a spring-clean. Typically, when my clients stop or severely limit their intake of wheat and dairy, they will lose inches from previously bloated areas, and may also find it easier to achieve their ideal weight. Remember, I'm not a slimming clinic or weight loss guru, I only advocate losing weight for health reasons.

In this frantic day and age, there is another element which I believe is extremely important: To look radiant, de-stressing is vital. The best facial cannot help you if you are clogged up with stress and worry.

be good to yourself

You may be unable to shift some of your worries and concerns; your life may be so full that for a while you have little choice but to drive yourself hard. If that sounds like you, make sure you still take time out for yourself. Have a massage, a long bath or an early night with freshly laundered, sweet-smelling sheets. These are all tactile experiences, and touch has remarkable healing qualities. Stroking the fur of a cat or dog has the power to lower your heart rate and increase the release of endorphins – the feel-good chemicals that are also found in abundance in chocolate. By extension, cuddling your partner has the same benefits – and is less fattening!

It's no coincidence that all the latest treatments at my clinic are applied with the touch of the fingertips. You need a minimum of products coupled, most importantly, with the therapeutic touch of your own hands. Use your fingers for cleansing, rather than cotton wool or a flannel. This approach offers the additional advantage that your hands will also benefit from the products you use, and are less likely to become an age give-away.

The skin is richly supplied with nerve endings. Stimulating your facial skin encourages the flow of oxygen-rich blood and nutrients into the muscles, and encourages the discharge of waste materials away from the tissues.

But do use a light touch – I don't believe in manhandling the skin. The lighter the touch, the better the therapy, as a heavier touch is more likely to disturb any underlying toxins which could then emerge as spots. When you saunter upstairs you don't need to tell your heart to make more blood, the instruction comes automatically from the parasympathetic nervous system. In the same way, a gentle touch on the face is enough to encourage the skin to embrace its own healing strategies.

Contained in this book are some of my greatest self-care tools for caring for your face. I'm a great believer in polishing (see page 13) rather than exfoliating; it's a more gentle method that gives your face a luminous glow without disturbing the underlying tissues. Water left in a hole in the ground will eventually stagnate, but running water always stays fresh. Your skin functions in the same way. If you polish your skin twice a day, your cells will never build up to the point where they stagnate, and you'll find that your skin starts to look more radiant.

beauty wisdom

The truth is that you don't need oodles of money to look beautiful, but you do need common sense. I'm going to be giving you lots of practical and inexpensive remedies distilled from experience and insights handed down through generations of my family. Naturally, as a teenager I sometimes resented my mother's home-spun approach to beauty care, where so many skin care products were made in the kitchen, using ingredients from the cupboard. But now I value such simplicity. It is in memory of my mother that I work hard to bring such practicality into other people's lives. When I first started my work as a therapist, people found me unusual: I was turning my back on fancy, expensive ingredients and modern chemicals, for my mother had taught me beauty wisdom.

As we age there is a tendency for our faces to put on weight, and because of the effect of gravity the excess tends to sag off the muscle, leading to a 'jowly' appearance. One of the best ways to combat this does not involve anything more complex than a carrot used to create an effective facial exercise. After every meal I try to eat one carrot, chewing each mouthful until it completely liquefies in my mouth. All this chewing tones the face naturally and you also benefit from the vitamin A the carrot contains, which acts as an antioxidant to help prevent your skin from becoming dry or rough. (Supplement this with one kiwi-fruit eaten daily, a tasty natural vitamin pill that contains vitamin C and potassium – which help lower high blood cholesterol and reduce the risk of cancer and heart disease.)

As an added tip, keep an eye on your bowel movements. It may not be a particularly pleasant or elegant subject to discuss, but you need to face up to the fact that if you are constipated you are going to suffer skin problems. Full stop. Forget that expensive feel-good potion you are considering buying, and focus instead on becoming regular by eating extra roughage and upping your fresh water intake. Encourage everything out and you'll prevent toxins from building up. This is all part of my no-nonsense approach to beauty care.

nature and nurture

I'm a natural therapist, and I believe it is always better to use natural therapies where possible, but in cases where more radical help is required I do sometimes condone a more focused intervention, and so I have included a *Nurture* section in this book which will give you the know-how to decide whether a specialized treatment is for you. Prevention is always better than cure, but if you have failed to prevent your skin from some irreversible aspect of deterioration you may find this section useful as a resource to help you choose a more invasive treatment.

I had one client who had several very deep lines around her mouth which were destroying her confidence. In her case we discussed using Botox – to paralyse the lines – and Restylane – to fill them in, and she decided that because of the severity of the problem that this would be a good solution. She went ahead, the lines were successfully reduced and she is now much happier. Likewise, I had a client with a lot of hair growth on her upper lip who decided that laser hair removal was the only way to tackle her problem.

Sometimes women may decide to have micro-pigmentation on their lips and eyes, which lasts for between three and five years and negates the need to waste time and money on daily make-up. Subtlety is key here. It's not for everyone, but for some people more intervention can be very useful.

My beauty philosophies have grown from a rich cultural background that combines traditional Eastern remedies, passed down through generations, with Western technology. Always remember, the key to beauty lies in good health and inner vitality. Beauty is more than skin deep.

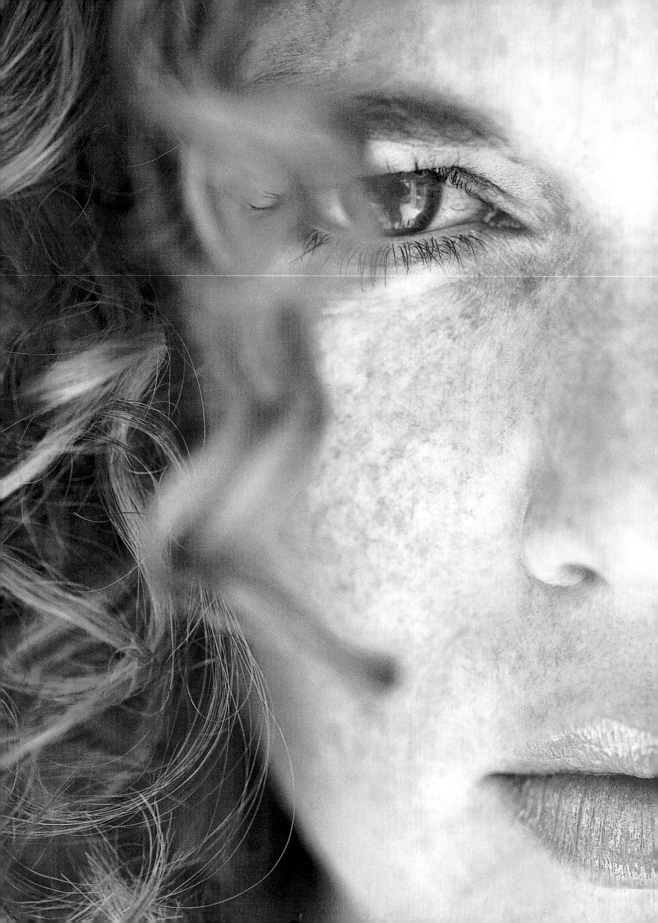

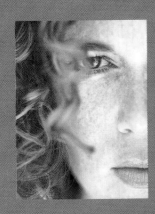

nature

Things you can do for your skin

your skin

We all lead busy lives, so the mainstay of my approach to skin care is helping women make better use of their time with an efficient facial care routine. My approach may have ancient Eastern roots, but it has to work in a fast-paced, modern context. My regimes are designed with simplicity in mind, and are never over-elaborate. If it doesn't feel natural and easy, I know that it's not going to become part of the way you do things. One of my fundamental beliefs is that a little goes a long way – spend a small amount of time on yourself and you will feel free to spend the rest on what you consider to be of most importance.

Problems with my own skin motivated me to develop my techniques: I know the effect that poorly performing skin has on self-esteem. I remember how my altered self-perception changed the way I related to other people, and how I stopped feeling comfortable in my own skin. I want to offer you a skin-care regimen that will make you feel and look fabulous within your time constraints. The essence of vitality is spending a small amount of time on yourself so that you can then attend to others. People are often not ill, but ill-balanced. The skin is my diagnostic starting point.

what is the skin?

The skin is your body's largest organ. It insulates and protects you and helps transmit sensory information from the outside to the inside. It isn't just an external covering, but a living, breathing organ as essential to your functioning as your heart, liver and kidneys.

It covers between 15 and 20 square feet, depending on your height and size. Every square inch contains 15 feet of blood vessels, 100 sweat glands, 1,500 sensory receptors and 12 feet of nerves.

The Epidermis

Skin has three layers. The top layer, or *epidermis*, is a thin protective barrier and is coated in a layer made up of dead skin cells which wear away at the rate of 10 billion cells every 24 hours. By the time we reach puberty, most of us have already damaged the baby soft skin we were born with following exposure to the sun. As you age, the tendency is for this layer to thicken as the natural skin-shedding process slows down, leaving your skin looking rather tired and pallid.

The Dermis

Just underneath the epidermis is the *dermis*, the highly active part of the skin. It contains the hair follicles, sweat glands, and collagen and elastin fibres which give the skin its elastic strength. Here, all those endless layers of cells are produced which are gradually exposed as they mature and move outwards to the skin's surface, eventually forming the protective layer on top. It is the dermis that absorbs moisturizers and gives the impression of plumped-up skin, as the cells swell for up to 12 hours, giving the illusion of youth.

But as you get older, the collagen and elastin fibres lose some of their elasticity; when this is coupled with gravity it leads to an unavoidable slackening of the skin. At puberty our pores widen and oil glands start working in response to male and female hormones, leading to acne.

Collagen

This is your skin's natural pre-tensioner, keeping the fabric of your skin in shape. Unfortunately, as we age its tightly organized mesh of fibres begins to break down. Instead of sitting neatly in a tight, regular pattern, the collagen fibres spread out and skin starts to look more baggy. The first lines are visible around the eyes and mouth, as these are the most over-worked part of our expressive apparatus. The collagen ages faster in these locations because of constant use.

Elastin

Collagen fibres contain elastin. This is the skin's natural Lycra, which helps the skin to stay snug and taut, and just like a pair of leggings washed in too-hot water which eventually fade and go baggy at the knees, so the elastin in our skin becomes less responsive. The chemical term for the equivalent response in skin is *oxidation*, and it is the result of too much sunshine, stretching through decades of facial expression, rough treatment with your hand towel, and an increasingly sluggish blood supply starving the skin of nutrition.

The Subcutis

The third layer of the skin is called the *subcutis* and is formed of fat which feeds and supports the upper layers. We tend to think of body fat as a bad thing, but remove the cushioning effect of the subcutis and we would look emaciated and unattractive, exposing the bed of muscle upon which the skin sits. As we age, much of the underlying fat is lost from the face, creating baggy necks and saggy jowls.

As we age, our skin ages with us. It gradually dries out and we develop freckles, age spots and broken capillaries. Our pores continue to enlarge and our facial colour becomes irregular. Some of the changes detailed here cannot be helped, but others will respond to intervention if you start early enough.

The most important thing you can do is understand your skin type and learn how to care for it. If you have a new car, you know it will break down if you don't put in oil, water and the appropriate lubricants. Failing to take it for regular services will soon see it lose peak performance. Your skin is just the same.

An Important Note About Your Neck

All my guidelines for facial skin care also apply to your neck, down to your breast bone. Your neck has no sebaceous glands and therefore makes no natural oil. If you overlook your neck and don't polish and moisturize it effectively, it will eventually look rough and pimply, and stand out as a signpost of your biological age.

your skin type

No two skins are the same. We inherit our basic skin type from our parents. This genetic disposition can be influenced by a range of other factors, and means that most people experience fluctuations in skin type as they age. Hormone changes create the most noticeable changes upon the skin's surface. Greasy skin during puberty, and dry skin during mid-life, are common side-effects of our maturing monthly cycle. Menstruation, pregnancy, using the contraceptive pill, the menopause and HRT all lead to changes in skin texture.

The skin is a signboard for our internal well-being; changes on the exposed face act as evidence of imbalance.

In addition, factors such as stress threshold, environment, diet, how effectively we digest our food and the cosmetics and skin care products we use on our skin all contribute to its eventual texture and moisture content. Other lesser factors include illness, changes in the weather, lack of exercise and anxiety.

Normal skin – that is, balanced skin that is neither too greasy nor too dry – is rare. And yet as babies we all start out with perfect skin. As children our skin is fairly thick, has invisible pores and feels velvety soft. Oil and moisture are evenly distributed across its surface and, when blotted with a tissue, there is evidence of a light moisture but no greasy residue. Modern diets, stress and over-exposure to the sun, along with hormone changes as we age, mean that this equilibrium is almost impossible to maintain.

However, that doesn't mean you have to abandon yourself to fate. There is a great deal you can do to harmonize your skin type, enhance problem skin and embrace a new luminescence.

First, you need to test the condition of your skin. Forget what you've been told in the past, your complexion may well have changed since then.

First, fold a tissue into a square and gently pat your forehead, turn it over and pat your cheeks. If the tissue shows no sign of oiliness or moisture, then your skin is too dry. If it appears to be covered in a film of grease, your skin is oily. If the tissue is slightly moist but does not appear greasy, your skin is well balanced.

Dry Skin

This is the most typical skin type, and eight in ten women will find their skin has become excessively dry at some point in their lives. You can tell if your skin is dry because it is likely to feel tight or look flaky. Trust yourself, you are the best judge of your own skin. Dryness is caused by a lack of sebum, the skin's natural oily lubricant, and leads to a thinning of the epidermis which means that tiny capillaries can often be seen through the translucent surface. Fine wrinkles and flaky dry patches are also often a problem. Skin of this type is unlikely to have enlarged pores.

This is skin that chaps easily, feels tight across the cheeks and forehead and is prone to itching and irritation.

The condition is likely to be worsened by exposure to detergents, sunshine, air-conditioning, poor diet, central heating and smoky environments.

The key to treating and caring for dry skin is encouraging it to normalize and retain more moisture.

Oily Skin

Oily skin is the result of excess of sebum production due to over-activity of the sebaceous glands caused by hormonal changes in the body, exacerbated in certain congested areas during the monthly cycle. The best way to assess how oily your skin is to use a small strip of sellotape placed on your skin. The marking on the tape shows exactly how oily the skin is. If the tape seems barely sticky and is covered in a thick residue when you pull it away, your skin is very oily.

Very oily skin is evidence of disharmony and stagnation in the skin. Characteristically, oily skin appears shiny, with visible open pores, a coarse texture and a sallow complexion. It is prone to clogging up and is therefore more vulnerable to pimples, blackheads and acne. The greasy surface is also a trap for dust and dirt, and regular washing is crucial if spots are not to form. There is also a tendency for make-up to slide off the skin. Oily skin tends to become a little less oily with age.

The advantage is that wrinkles are less common on oily skins, and so this sort of skin looks younger longer.

A Note About the Mysterious T-zone

The T-zone is a myth conjured up by people who think cosmetically, rather than holistically. It is nothing more than a central panel of oily skin, on the forehead, nose and chin – features which due to their prominence need most protection from the sebaceous glands.

So-called 'combination' skin is another name for the same zone, where over-active sebaceous glands create an oily panel. I don't believe in using different products to treat this area. It is far more beneficial to treat the whole face the same – in time, the over-oily centre will rectify itself.

Normal Skin

This is shorthand for skin that is more dry than oily. You are fortunate if you have drier skin, it is oily skin that creates a lot more problems. And while dry or normal skin benefits from stimulation, oily skin is very easily over-stimulated.

Basic Tips for Caring for Your Skin Type

Dry Skin

Tone before moisturizing with rose water (avoid toners containing alcohol, which have a drying action). You will benefit from an oil-based moisturizer. Because sunshine dries the skin still further, do not venture outside without a high-factor sunscreen applied to all exposed areas. Choose skin products that contain cucumber, evening primrose oil, arnica, lavender and camomile. This is skin that must never be left unprotected. I'm against heavy night creams; better to use a lighter version so the skin is encouraged to work for itself.

Oily Skin

The oily surface is a magnet for dust, so regular careful cleaning with soap and water is very important. You can also use an alcohol-based toner, which will refresh the skin and dry it out slightly, but avoid astringent lotions which will spur the sebaceous glands into producing yet more oil. The toner doesn't close the pores, rather it plumps the skin to give a more even-textured appearance and strengthens the skin's naturally protective acid mantle. Because you don't want to add yet more moisture to your face, avoid heavy oil-based moisturizers and opt instead for a light moisturizing milk designed for oily skin with added sunscreen – but remember that although we all need to cleanse the skin, we don't all need to use moisturizer. If your skin is still excessively oily, experiment without using moisturizer for a week (still use a sunscreen). If you over-moisturize oily skin you are preventing the skin from working for itself and finding a natural sebaceous balance. Never use heavy night creams on oily skin.

Choose skin-care products that contain calendula, chestnut, witch hazel, aloe vera or burdock.

Combination Skin

Wash as usual. Avoid using an alcohol-based toner. Instead, use rose water or, for a refreshing spritz which will encourage blood to the surface, splash your face with cold water. Avoid using moisturizer on the oily T-zone; instead, apply it judiciously to the drier areas only. Use a light sunscreen all over the face. Identifying the different types of skin in your face and caring for them differently is really worth the extra few seconds of attention each day, as your facial tone and texture will appear more consistent as a result.

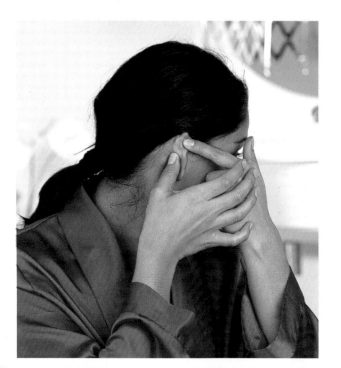

Normal Skin

Don't let dead cells build up; encourage the circulation so your skin does not stagnate; eat the right foods, and drink enough water.

Facial routines should always start with the neck, and include the jawline and behind the ear to activate the lymph glands.

Treat your face to a weekly massage (see Facial Lymphatic Drainage Massage, page 103).

routines for all types

Skin is an organic, living thing that is constantly changing its nature in response to diet, hormones and the weather. Look at the pattern of your lifestyle to determine how best to care for your skin. I want to empower you to understand the fundamentals: what your skin is trying to say and how best to care for it. If the weather is getting cold and you're going to be outside, use a more protective therapy including a nourishing cream. If you are using central heating and staying mostly inside, drink plenty of water to keep your skin from drying out, and use a lighter moisturizer. Take control of your looks. Knowledge is power in your own hands.

When it comes to your daily facial-care routine, simplicity is imperative. If you attempt to follow some enormously complex routine with countless products to open and close, the truth is that you're going to stop doing it after a few weeks. Instead, I'm going to give you a no-nonsense guide for caring for your skin which makes sense, is easy to follow and works at a deeper level to maintain the quality of your skin.

Daytime skin-care is all about protection against dehydration and pollution. At night, your skin needs to rest, recuperate and regenerate.

The Truth about Cleansing

We all need to keep our skin clean, it's the number one priority for your face, and you do need to do it twice a day, in the morning and at night. But your routine needs to vary slightly depending on the time of day, because your face is alternately immersed in two quite different environments.

While you are asleep your skin continues to release sebum through the pores which accumulate on the surface, while dead skin cells are being shed as the body undergoes night-time repair work.

During the day your face has to contend with the addition of environmental debris which sticks to its surface. Pollution, dust, pollen and smoke make up a 21st-century mask which, along with the make-up you put there during the course of the day, you certainly don't want to take to bed with you. If it is left on the surface of the skin overnight it slows down the repair process and prevents your skin from breathing.

The night-time clean is of primary importance. In the morning you can get away with a swipe with a damp flannel if pressed for time, but do make the time for a thorough cleanse in the evening.

Everything I am going to tell you applies from your cleavage upwards. The skin on your neck can be a real give-away, and if you want to wear low-cut tops you owe it to yourself to care for all exposed skin with due attention.

Should I Use Soap or Cleanser?

There's a lot of nonsense talked about soap. It's simply not true that you need to spend money on expensive cleansers in order to clean your face and be kind to your skin. Washing with (the right) soap is an extremely effective way to remove dirt and bacteria from your skin, although it is rapidly going out of fashion. However, providing that your skin is healthy, you rinse off all the residue and moisturize afterwards, this is a no-nonsense way of washing.

Never use perfumed soaps – these are entirely unnecessary and can irritate the skin. Avoid harsh soaps – these are too alkaline and so disturb the naturally acidic surface of the skin. Instead, buy pH-balanced soaps which don't strip the skin's natural moisture or leave your face feeling like a taut mask.

Remember that one of the most important parts of your cleansing routine is rinsing off the soap or cleanser you have used, or you'll have created an emulsion of dirt mixed with a nice layer of soapy food for bacteria to feed on.

Don't use really hot water, you risk weakening the small capillaries near the skin's surface until they eventually break. Cold water is good for a spritz by itself, but it won't emulsify soap or dissolve dirt and dead skin cells. I recommend using water that feels warm rather than hot; this will also help to get the circulation flowing.

Building up a rich lather of soap will help slough away all the debris on the skin's surface.

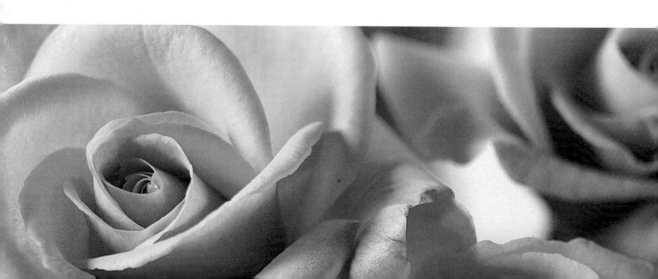

How to Wash

1 Massage the soap thoroughly all over your face and don't forget your neck, under your chin, the sides of your nose, your eyebrows and your chin. Wash it away with plenty of water. If you have time, repeat the process, before using some cold water to close any open pores.

2 If you have blackheads or congested skin on your nose, chin or forehead, wrap a flannel around your finger, wipe it across a bar of soap and use a moderate pressure to make small circular movements around the affected area. Rinse and repeat.

If you are prone to dry or sensitive skin, you may find your face feels tight when you use soap and you may be better off using a cleansing lotion with added moisturizer or a foaming cleanser without soap.

As a general rule, choose:

For dry/mature skin	cream cleanser
Normal skin	lotion cleanser
Oily skin	foaming or gel-based cleanser

Alternatively, try my favoured traditional method, which sounds unusual but actually makes perfect sense and is absolutely the best way to wash mature skin, skin prone to acne, or sensitive skin. Apply a light film of almond oil or unrefined vegetable oil, such as sunflower, all over your neck and face. Rub it in gently with the balls of your fingertips and leave for one minute. Then remove with a pad of dampened cotton wool. The oil will dissolve all the grime and build-up, without stripping the skin of its protective film.

Some people say you should only dab your face with a towel, but I think this is a lost opportunity. Rubbing your face very gently is an effective way to slough off any lingering dead skin cells. A sideways motion is better than rubbing up and down, as this can encourage the muscles to sag.

Read your own skin: If it looks taut and tight after washing, you need to try another approach.

Cleansing Routines

Always start at the neck and linger a little longer on the drier areas rather than over-stimulating the oilier areas. Use a light touch, if you use too much pressure and there is toxicity lurking beneath the skin, you may provoke an outbreak of spots. All skin types benefit from a light cleanser.

Removing Make-up

The only time to use a heavier cleanser is when you are wearing a lot of make-up, in which case my advice is to first loosen the make-up with a dab of almond oil applied with your finger and dabbed off with a dry tissue prior to cleansing. There is no need to buy an expensive make-up remover.

Dry Skin

Cleanse the driest part of your skin first, and for longer, to help loosen the dead cells.

Oily Skin

Before you cleanse, use a cleansing wipe or a muslin cloth, or moisten a strong three-ply tissue, to lightly rub off excess oil and dead skin cells before you cleanse. Then, very lightly cleanse the oily areas with a light cleanser, avoiding the urge to over-stimulate the skin. The temptation is to think that because there is more oil you should focus on removing it. But that will only stimulate the sebaceous glands and cause them to produce more oil. Oily areas tend to have a build-up of dead cells because of this over-activity.

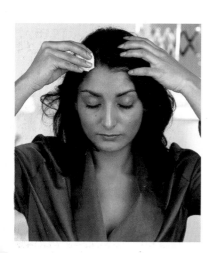

Normal Skin

For maintaining nicely-balanced skin, remember: The lighter the touch, the better the therapy. Start with the neck and move up the face. Never put too much pressure on the delicate facial skin when cleansing. Choose a light, pH-balanced cleanser. Even better is to choose a cleansing wipe – the slightly abrasive nature of the wipe gives a light exfoliation, though it should be used very lightly.

Polishing

The polishing routine is very important and is a keystone of my philosophy. You can use a gentle polisher twice a day as an ideal way of refining the skin's texture, improving its circulation and clearing the pores. Polishing is neither a scrub nor an exfoliation, rather it is a much gentler way of giving your face a radiant glow. You wouldn't buff oak furniture with coarse granules, as contained in a lot of the so-called facial scrubs on the market today.

Polishing the skin may sound like a strange concept, but people polish their cars, ornaments and anything else they hold dear and want to look shiny and new. I believe the body deserves just as much special care. What's more, it's extremely good for your skin.

Polishing stimulates the skin, removes dead skin cells and leaves your face feeling baby-soft, with a healthy glow. It stops the skin building up unwanted layers, and stimulates blood flow to the skin's surface without over-abrading it.

This invigorating, de-clogging process helps the skin to function properly and helps its excretory activities to continue effectively. Another benefit of this form of touch is the way it stimulates cell reproduction deeper in the dermis. But you mustn't be too vigorous. If you are too rough you can damage the underlying tissue and create broken capillaries.

The days of cleansers/toners are numbered. Oil and polishing are key to the new revolution, and things I was taught as a child by my mother. On Sunday mornings in the bathroom she would show me how to polish my skin. As a teenager I was prone to severe acne. My mother was a 'compounder' – one of the early pharmacists – and she would make me up a custom treatment which I will share with you here.

My Mother's Polisher

Mix a tablespoon of ghee (melted butter) with a tablespoon of milk and rub into a small bowl of gram (chickpea) flour. Leave overnight and then apply to the skin with a gentle polishing motion, to nourish and clean. This recipe is perfect for any skin type. My mother called it *Chaamak*, which in Gujarati means 'it will bring radiance' and she had been taught this by my grandmother, who was ahead of her time.

Simple Polisher

If you're in a rush, mix two teaspoons of oatmeal with one teaspoon of almond oil. Oatmeal helps to slough off the cells without being abrasive.

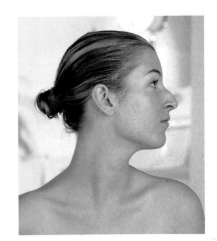

Polishing is a skin-care process that helps to normalize and balance the skin, irrespective of skin type. Polishing stimulates nerve endings, lymphatic circulation and the capillary networks. Exfoliants and scrubs are too harsh for the skin. Polishing is a much gentler approach, and you must apply with a light touch. Deal with wrinkles at the polishing stage by lingering over wrinkled areas to encourage blood circulation.

How to Polish

First of all, dampen your neck and face. Take a generous amount of polisher on the palm of your hand and, using your fingertips, gently stroke rather than scour your skin. You want to work very lightly all over, including under the eyes, behind the ears, and on top of the eyelids. The idea is to gently massage your skin in an upward direction with a light touch. There is no separate beauty routine necessary for the eye as long as you are gentle, and polishing will can help with dark circles and puffy eyes. Spend about two minutes very lightly making light upward circular motions with the tips of your fingertips all over your face. Then pat with luke-warm water. Dry by patting with a towel, and you are ready for moisturizing.

Irrespective of your skin type, polishing will have a balancing effect.

Toning

Toners are water-based products which may contain alcohol. They were devised to counter-balance the effect of cleansers which could upset the pH balance while cleaning the skin of debris and make-up, and are now largely out of date.

I'm a great believer in hydrotherapy: The best toner is cold water, splashed on after polishing and before moisturizing so that the skin is left moist and slightly tighter. The function is to close the pores and to increase circulation, which helps accelerate the delivery of nutrients and the removal of toxins.

Coconut Toner

Grate fresh coconut and a drop of milk to use as a toner.

The Importance of Moisturizer

Moisturizer is very important. If you place an apple outside for a few days, the skin will gradually wrinkle as it loses moisture. Our skin behaves in the same way. Moisturizer is important, but don't overload the skin.

Our skin makes its own natural moisturizer, an unappetizing sounding mixture of sebum and sweat which is dispersed in a thin layer over our body through our pores. It exists to maintain the skin's softness by maintaining the moisture level in the outermost layer of skin cells. The oil acts as a waterproof barrier which halts the evaporative process, while the sweat provides the skin with an acidic buffer to stop it coming under attack from bacteria.

Moisturizing creams mimic this oil/water mixture in an emulsion of varying proportions. Unfortunately, many facial moisturizers are too heavy, and night creams too rich. The tendency to over-moisturize undermines the skin's capacity to keep itself taut. It's really not true that increasing the intensity of our beauty care by spending a lot of money on rich creams is the best option. Far better is to use common sense and simplicity, cleaning your face and then locking in the moisture with the lightest moisturizer possible for your skin type. Moisturizers should only be used to *assist* the skin's function, not replace it.

Choose a product which is 'oil free' and also non-comedogenic or non-acnegenic, as these are less likely to lead to blackheads.

A lot of nonsense is talked by cosmetic companies who add an array of ingredients to make us part with more money that we should. A product cannot get rid of wrinkles, neither can a potion in a pot eradicate years of neglect. What they can do is add water to skin and seal in the skin's own moisture. This plumps up skin cells for up to 12 hours (which is why you should moisturize twice a day). This is especially important for older skin because its elastin and collagen are less effective at retaining moisture, especially if you are a smoker or have sun damage. Well-hydrated skin feels comfortable and helps you look healthy.

Instead of trying an expensive cream, try one of the most effective and mildest of all moisturizers – unrefined nut and seed oil found in a healthfood shop – for a fraction of the cost. The mother of a friend of mine was 80 years old and had the most perfect supple skin. When I asked her for her secret, she said for 40 years she had applied a few dabs of olive oil to her skin every night before bed, a habit begun during the war when shop-bought moisturizer was an unattainable luxury. She proved you really don't need it. Natural oils gently soften and lubricate the skin, while the vitamin E they contain helps to counter the effect of over-exposure to sunshine. Use sparingly after cleansing, or, for an all-over treat, cover yourself in a layer before showering and pat dry afterwards.

Apply your chosen moisturizing oil or cream to slightly damp skin twice a day, immediately after washing or splashing your face. The layer of fats that are deposited from the product on the surface of your skin trap a fine layer of water next to the skin.

Remember, moisturizers produce no permanent change. They only make your skin look better by making it look plumper. It's a cosmetic change, but makes a difference to the way you feel about yourself.

If you are using a separate sunscreen, apply it at least quarter of an hour after your moisturizer.

Use a small amount of moisturizer so you don't overwhelm your skin and completely upset your body's natural production of sebum.

Always use your hands to **apply** products to your face. I'm a great believer in the healing properties of touch, so dump your cotton wool pads and use your own fingertips to massage in moisturizer using a light upward stroke to work against gravity.

People make a big deal about moisturizing, but I am a great believer in simplicity. Know your skin and follow the basics and you won't run into trouble. The lighter the moisturizer, the better. Don't overload your skin. Apply moisturizer all over your face, including under the eyes. If the moisturizer is as light as it should be, it will be appropriate even for the delicate eye area.

Oily Skin

Even if your skin is very oily you must always use moisturizer to encourage it to normalize. Choose lighter moisturizers – these are oil in water (heavier ones are water in oil). Put a few dots on your face and keep rubbing with the balls of your fingers, very lightly, until it is absorbed into the skin.

Dry Skin

This is skin that is losing moisture at an accelerated rate or where the dead cells are building up on the skin's surface. Dry skins benefit from a nourishing cream which feeds them, but don't choose one that is so heavy it overwhelms the skin. Products containing glycerine and macadamia nut oil help the skin hold on to moisture without being too heavy.

Dry skin needs more protection, but a common mistake is thinking you need to use a heavy moisturizer. You may have a lot of latent toxins under the skin, and when you use a rich moisturizer it merely seals the pores and prevents the skin from breathing, which can result in spots. Follow a twice-daily polishing routine.

Flaky Skin

If your skin is flaky you may have a skin disorder which needs separate treatment. Dry skin does not usually flake, it simply fails to hold on to moisture and dead cells and needs additional lubrication. Flaky skin is evidence of an imbalance of moisture in the cells. Polishing can help, but you may need additional skin care.

On the driest of dry skin, use almond oil to moisturize. Within three weeks the skin will have normalized.

Normal Skin

A light moisturizer is a must. You might have the healthiest skin, but if you don't moisturize it will be prone to wrinkles.

Alpha Hydroxyl Acid

Some moisturizers contain Alpha Hydroxyl Acid (a naturally occurring chemical extracted from milk, sugar cane, grapes and citrus fruits). The acid accelerates the sloughing-off of dead skin cells by dissolving the 'glue' that holds the dead cells together. If you must, use only once a day, preferably in the morning. However, I'm sceptical about the efficacy of AHA when mixed into moisturizer. It makes a more effective maintenance tool when used in over-the-counter concentrations of not more than 10 per cent, and can then be considered a safe skin refresher which can help you achieve smoother, clearer, less wrinkle-free skin. However, do not confuse AHA solutions with AHA peels. These much higher doses burn off a layer of the skin. Bear in mind that using even a mild AHA solution can cause skin irritation, redness and itching if you have sensitive skin.

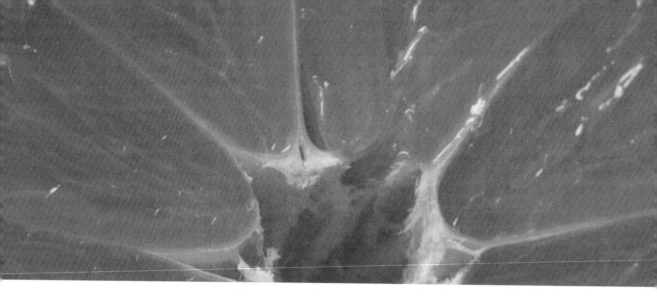

feeding your skin from within

Many beauty advisers concentrate only on external skin-care, but your skin's well-being is absolutely dependent on good internal nourishment and lifestyle choices. Here are some simple – but essential – methods of helping your skin reach its radiant potential.

Eat a healthy diet: Failing to eat enough nutrients leads to poorly nourished skin, prone to sallowness and disorders. Good digestion is also important if your body is to benefit from the nutrients in the good-quality food you do eat.

Drink plenty of water: A low fluid intake dehydrates the skin's cells, making them appear dry and more prone to disorders.

Exercise regularly: Too little exercise can have adverse effects on the various hormones which the skin needs to regenerate itself, including insulin (which regulates blood fats and sugar) and oestrogen (which keeps cells plump).

Live a stress-free lifestyle: Being over-stressed produces hormones that narrow arteries and encourage cholesterol to build up.

Do not smoke: Smoking narrows arteries and encourages them to clog with cholesterol, reducing blood flow to the skin.

Get sufficient sleep: Broken sleep or too few hours at a stretch stop the skin from healing and growing. It is during our sleeping hours that we produce the highest levels of the hormones that encourage skin to heal, with the greatest benefits during the six, seventh and eighth hours of sleep.

Medical Indications Leading to Troubled Skin

Reduced production of certain hormones can lead to skin disorders. See your doctor if you are concerned about the following:

Under-active thyroid: Skin looks dry and feels cold, eyebrows and lashes fall out.

Reduced oestrogen (as at the menopause): Skin thins, looks less plump and appears dry or lined. HRT and eating naturally-occurring plant oestrogens can help.

Underproduction of insulin: The onset of diabetes leads to sallow, grey skin as arteries are narrowed by a rapid build-up of cholesterol.

Fluid retention, or medical conditions that interfere with the body's ability to remove tissue fluid, leading to bloating, can also lead to skin problems. Causes can be food sensitivity, premenstrual syndrome, pregnancy, or heart or kidney or liver disease.

signs of ageing

When you are born you are wrapped in a blemish-free coating. You are like a Christmas present that is perfectly gift-wrapped, with creases only where they are necessary to allow a smooth fit and flexibility. Over time your skin becomes like a parcel that has been handled too many times. The wrapping begins to break down and show the signs of wear and tear that express its history. By the end of its life-cycle, the formerly smooth surface has become crimped after all that bending and folding and stretching. But unlike a parcel, which would be damaged after just a few days of such treatment, your facial skin is amazingly resilient. It's only after two decades or so that any sign at all of age begins to show upon its surface.

There is nothing you can do to stop the changes in your skin. From your mid-twenties onwards it begins to lose its smooth texture, firm tone and uniform colour. The skin's support structure collapses, and wrinkles appear. Reduced blood flow means the skin isn't able to nourish cells or discourage the build-up of waste toxins. This breakdown happens to us all at a pace determined by our genes, but influenced by environmental factors including smoking, poor diet, sun damage, stress and neglectful care. Exposure to the ultraviolet radiation in sunshine, the chemicals in cigarettes and atmospheric pollution hasten the creation of free radicals, minute particles that accelerate tissue degeneration (see page 23).

Even if your skin has suffered I believe it's never too late to help redress the effects of the ageing process. This is not to say you should crave an ageless face. Your face is part of your personality, it carries evidence of wisdom, confidence and experience. The trouble only starts when you lose confidence in your appearance because the changes are too radical or are accelerating too rapidly. Your skin does not have to show your age if you put certain routines and habits into practice early enough.

The basic guide skin-care guide which every mother would do well to teach her daughters does not involve lots of complicated potions, but common sense. The best way to care for your skin is a process of EFP – eating, flushing, polishing. That is, choosing a healthy nutrient-rich diet, flushing your system with lots of water – a minimum of eight glasses a day – and using my polishing routine (see page 14).

Over-exposure to the sun and a lack of basic skin cleansing will make you appear to age more quickly, and without vitamins, minerals, amino-acids and enzymes the skin will deteriorate.

Free Radicals

We burn oxygen to power our bodies, but just like burning fossil fuels, there is a damaging by-product: free radicals. In small quantities these are helpful as they help fight off infection, but they also attack our own cells in a process that is the body's equivalent of rusting. This process of oxidation attacks the cells like rust attacks untreated metal. The proteins are corrupted, the membranes are torn, the cellular fats turn rancid and even the genetic component of the cells is vulnerable. When we smoke, breathe in environmental pollutants or spend time in the sunshine, we absorb huge quantities of free radicals from outside our bodies.

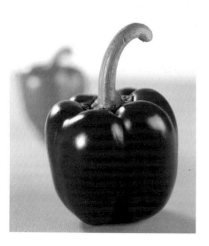

The reason free radicals have this damaging effect is that they are molecules missing an electron which they attempt to steal from a healthy cell. This process can be neutralized by eating food rich in antioxidants. These contain compounds that have electrons to spare and ensure that the free radicals are returned to normal.

Choose foods full of vitamins C and E and beta-carotene – the substance the body uses to create vitamin A. Carotenes are part of the colour systems in plants, so as a rule choose richly coloured foods: broccoli, orange and red peppers, apricots, cabbage, tomatoes, carrots. To work their best the antioxidants need certain minerals, so you should also supplement your diet with nuts. Brazil nuts are best, they contain selenium which is an important part of the natural antioxidant system.

Why We Age

Over the years many theories have been suggested as to why our bodies age. The quest for this knowledge has become the new grail of the pharmaceutical and skin-care industries: Until you unravel the intricacies of the process you can't hope to reverse it. For years it was thought that ageing was the result of a lifetime of unexpelled toxins building up in the body, or because of wear and tear on the body's tissues or because of a decline in our immune system, making us more vulnerable to attack. It is now known that ageing occurs at a cellular level.

Every cell contains chromosomes which are made up of DNA, a molecule that contains the code for making a human being. As we grow during childhood, the DNA makes a copy of itself in each cell before splitting into two new cells. Once we are fully grown, the process slows down and the DNA only makes enough new copies to replace those that are damaged or that die from time to time. But unfortunately, when the DNA copies itself it gets a little smaller each time. When we are children the process doesn't affect the quality of the copy because the DNA includes some 'padding' which can be missed off without causing a problem. But when the replication takes place as we grow older, we no longer have any of this padding left over for the inexact process of biological photocopying, and tiny fragments of genetic information themselves start disappearing. Each new cell division compounds the effect.

As the perfect blueprint is corrupted in this way, our cell processes – hair, body, skin, muscles – start to age. It is our genetic inheritance that determines how quickly we begin to see this ageing. Some people have less of the spare padding than others, or replicate more quickly.

Scientists are currently working on techniques to genetically alter human cells with an enzyme that will indefinitely create extra cell padding so that the vital genetic information does not deteriorate over time.

Perhaps one day all this will come to fruition, but for now the best you can do is care for your skin in an attempt to limit the ravages of the natural ageing process.

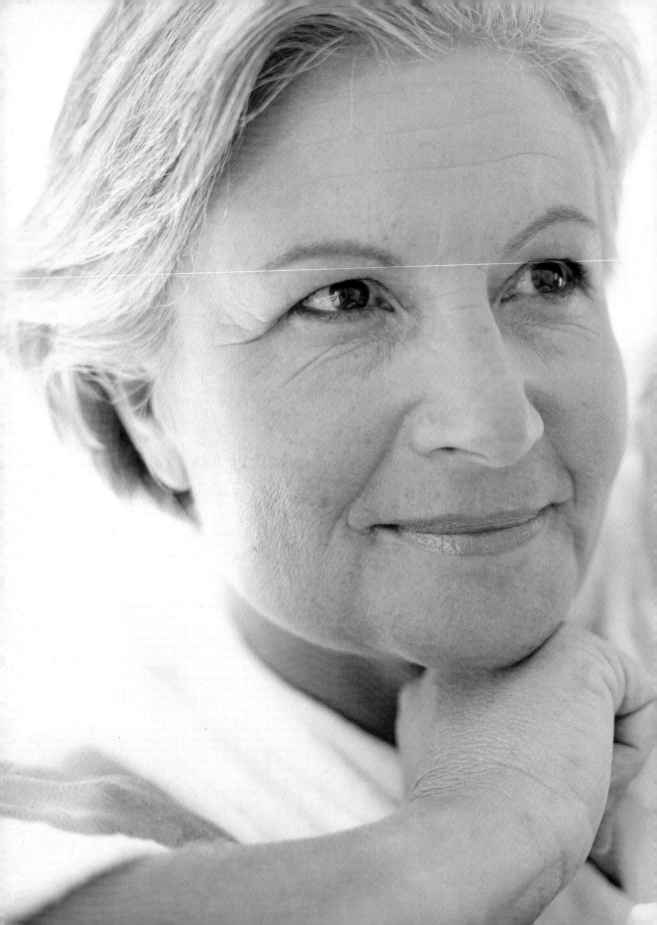

How to Slow Down Ageing

● A study completed last year by Imperial College London's Care of the Elderly Department, found that looking old for your age may have as much to do with chemicals in your blood as with your way of life. It's possible that small blood vessels are damaged by high cholesterol, making the skin look more wrinkled.

● The researchers also found that men who look older than their years had high levels of haemoglobin, the pigment in red blood cells that carries oxygen. The suggestion is that this can make blood thicker and more sluggish.

● Surprisingly, the study discovered that looking older was not related to alcohol consumption or level of success at work. Yet genetics, lifestyle and exercise can all influence cholesterol levels, a contributing factor.

● Other research, conducted in Edinburgh, comprised a 10-year study which concluded that genes were only 25 per cent responsible for youthful appearance – our behaviour was the chief factor behind the other 75 per cent.

● Regular exercise can slow ageing. Texas scientists found a 22-week programme of walking for 70-year-olds reversed decades of declining lung function, improved posture and cut the risk of age-related disability.

● A positive mental outlook can make a difference. Doctors have observed that depressed patients tend to have furrowed brows and more wrinkles. You can wipe years off your face by tackling depression and changing your natural expression (see page 113).

● Sleep is a factor because body tissues regenerate more efficiently when we're sleeping. Sleep deprivation causes a stress response that can affect the heart and small blood vessels in the skin. The skin under the eyes is particularly sensitive to this.

● Smoking affects the skin by reducing the amount of collagen produced, leading to a lack of suppleness and increasing the amount of wrinkles. In several studies of twins, the non-smoker was observed to look much younger than the smoker.

● People are increasingly aware of the link between over-exposure to sunshine and skin cancer, but few realize that skin cancer is the final result of accelerated ageing of skin tissue. In comparisons of twins who live in different climates, the one exposed to more sunlight always looked dramatically older.

Wrinkles

Wrinkles are a sign that skin is losing its elasticity. Permanent creases are a sign that the collagen fibres have undergone a change which undermines their ability to erase the temporary lines made by habitual patterns of expression. At the same time, changing hormone levels leads to a drop in the skin's oil and moisture levels. This compounds the problem, as water is required to keep collagen pliable.

The first signs of ageing are often seen on the neck, hands and around the eyes, so it's vital to pay special attention to these areas. Exfoliating can be too harsh; instead, polish your skin regularly, using upward strokes to defeat gravity. This will speed up the process of shedding the dead cells that make skin look dull.

The most important element in sustaining younger-looking skin is aiding the skin in its process of dead cell removal. Your skin is changing, but it can appear to be deteriorating faster if you let the dead skin cells accumulate, giving a congested grey cast to your face. Use a gentle facial polish once a day for three weeks, then weekly, to encourage the skin to slough off old cells.

Youth Polisher

Mix two teaspoons of double cream with two heaped teaspoons of fine oatmeal. Rub into the skin with a very light action using the balls of your fingers. Avoid using too firm a pressure on any one particular spot.

If you really want to stop the onset of wrinkles and you smoke: stop. The toxins in cigarette smoke have a devastating effect on our skin. The blood of a smoker has a high level of carbon monoxide, a poisonous gas that takes the place of all the oxygen we need. Smoking deprives the skin's cells of their oxygen diet, with the result that a smoker's skin looks heavy, prematurely lined and has a greyish, oxygen-starved pallor.

Anti-wrinkle Remedies

- Try to become aware of your expression. If you habitually use the same muscles when your face is resting, perhaps wrinkling your forehead or furrowing your brow, you will habituate that expression and wrinkles will result. Try to consciously relax the muscles to encourage the skin to stay smooth.

- Use a mild, oil-based cleanser to avoid stripping the skin of its natural oil and moisture. Remove cleanser with a damp cloth. Alternatively, almond oil applied to your lips and the skin around your mouth nightly will help to keep the area supple and line-free. Almond oil is also a terrific facial cleanser and moisturizer.

- Boost your vitamin C count by including some fresh fruit and vegetables in every meal. Ensure you are eating a protein-rich diet.

- Stimulate your facial circulation by using small pinching movements whenever you have a spare moment. Increasing the blood supply will nourish and help repair tissue damage.

- A stabilizing face mask is also a good way to help soothe skin prone to wrinkling or sensitivity. Mix one teaspoon of double cream with two teaspoons of water, a pinch of salt and one heaped teaspoon of gram (chickpea) flour, which can be found in a healthfood shop or Asian supermarket. Mix into a thick paste, apply and leave for 10 minutes before rinsing off.

- If you want to reduce the appearance of fine lines for a special occasion, firm the skin prior to applying make-up by gently beating the white of an egg and applying to the skin for 15 minutes. Personally I don't like the smell, but this is an effective treatment.

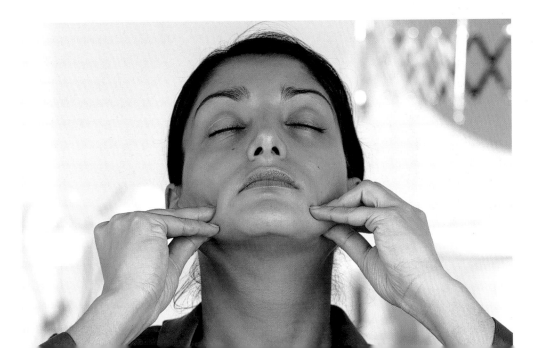

facial hair

As we mature, our hormone levels alter, and increasing testosterone (a perfectly common side-effect of maturation in women) can lead to the odd stray hair growing on our faces, particularly under our chin. This can be a bit disturbing at first, but it's really nothing to worry about.

If you have just a couple of hairs, they can be physically removed by shaving with a thin lubricant layer of soap, or by plucking them out once or twice a week when they have just emerged (keep an extra pair of tweezers in your make-up bag so you can whip one out if you notice it). If you prefer, you can melt away the visible hair with a chemical depilatory cream every four weeks. Alternatively you may want to consider electrolysis or laser treatment (see pages 160 and 165) to remove them permanently, particularly if you have more than a couple.

Dealing with Your Upper Lip

By the age of 65, four women in every 10 have a moustache above their upper lip. If yours bothers you, bear in mind that plucking is not realistic, given all these tiny hairs. Waxing or depilation, which dissolves the protein structure of the hair, may be your best bet for semi-permanent removal. Melted wax or cold-wax tapes are placed on the skin and the hairs become embedded in the wax as it hardens. Pull off the wax and the hairs come too, though they grow back in two weeks or so. Some damage to the follicle will occur, which means that over time the moustache may thin as the hairs reduce in quantity. Waxing can lead to the skin becoming red, so conduct the treatment the day *before* any big event.

Alternatively, rather than removing the hair, you could bleach your moustache to reduce its appearance. This is particularly appropriate if you have dark hair and simply want to reduce its impact. Bleaching agents are often potent chemicals, so only buy a preparation specifically designed for the upper lip because of the proximity to your mouth. Moustache hair is commonly bleached using a mixture of hydrogen peroxide and a mild alkaline such as ammonia. This treatment is best sought in a salon, but you can buy mild bleaching kits from chemists. Make sure you wash thoroughly afterwards and moisturize *immediately*.

What to Do About Your Chin

All healthy women produce small amounts of testosterone, but its influence is normally obscured by oestrogen. As we age, oestrogen levels begin to drop slightly and we begin to notice the influence of the male hormone. As a result, the odd follicle starts pushing up a thicker hair than the soft, barely-visible down that we have throughout childhood.

The best way to sort out those stray hairs on your chin is by plucking, waxing or using a depilatory cream. Depilatory creams are strongly alkaline (skin and hair are naturally very acidic), so they effectively dissolve the hair. Some women find it quicker to shave off the hair. This is fine if it suits you, and shaving certainly will NOT make the hair grow back thicker, that's a myth. However, because the hair is being sliced off at an angle at the surface of the skin it may appear more obvious. It will also grow out very quickly, which means you will have to shave every couple of days if you're bothered by the way the hair looks. Far better is to wax, pluck or depilate chemically. If you can afford it, consider electrolysis, but do bear in mind you may need several treatments, and that it can lead to scarring if your clinician is not competent.

skin disorders and blemishes, and how to treat them

Acne

This chronic inflammatory skin disease, called *acne vulgaris* in full, is often misunderstood. Most people think it affects only pubescent teenagers and can't understand why they should be suffering later in life. The answer is stress – the primary cause of first-time acne in women in their twenties. Seventy per cent of people will grow out of acne, but this simply doesn't happen to everyone and some people will suffer throughout their adult lives. It can also be a symptom of premenstrual syndrome. Doctors take the condition seriously because of the psychological harm it can inflict, as well as the scarring that can result. So the first place to go if you are suffering is your doctor, who should be sympathetic to the condition. Five per cent of women in their forties suffer from acne, so if you are one of them you are certainly not alone.

What Causes Acne?

Acne is caused when the oil gland becomes overly sensitive to the male hormone that we all, male or female, have in our bodies. This causes more sebum (the skin's own oil) to be produced in the hair follicle, creating greasy skin. In addition to this, acne causes a change in the cells that line the hair follicles: usually they die and are flushed on to the skin's surface, keeping the follicle open, but with acne, instead of being loosened ready for expulsion, the dead cells become sticky and attach themselves to the inside of the canal. Eventually the pore becomes completely blocked, just as in a blackhead (see page 32). It enlarges as the blockage is mixed with bacteria. If it's a deep blockage, the skin is pushed up above the stale oil that has collected. With nowhere else to go the oil pushes down into the hair canal, where it stagnates and absorbs water. The follicle by now is completely sealed, and the hair canal inflates like a tiny balloon under the skin's surface as bacteria start to multiply, leading to inflammation. The body senses this and white blood cells arrive in the follicle to kill the inflammation, creating pus which, eventually, under pressure, bursts on to the skin's surface, emptying the follicle.

Sore red lumps which last for a couple of weeks on the skin's surface are caused when the blockage is so severe that the pus cannot emerge up onto the skin, and instead bursts inwards. Squeezing spots can also lead to this internal bursting, and scarring can be the result.

How to Treat Acne

Although you cannot cure acne – the biological switch that is believed to cause it has to switch itself off – you can help reduce the severity of attacks and the likelihood of reinfection.

Do not touch or squeeze the spots.

Vitamin B_5 and vitamin B_6 play essential roles in maintaining healthy skin and fighting infection. Taking a daily multi-vitamin that contains the recommended dosage of all vitamins is a good idea.

Vitamin B_5 cream applied to the skin can also help. In one trial, individuals with moderate acne saw improvements after two months of daily use.

Eat a healthy diet, and limit your consumption of wheat and dairy products, sugar, processed food, salt, fatty foods and red meat. Try to eat two pieces of fresh fruit a day, stick to rice instead of pasta, and choose vegetables and salad, live yoghurt, garlic, seeds and nuts, fresh fish and free-range eggs.

Drink plenty of fresh water – eight glasses a day sounds a lot, but it will help to keep the system flushed and clean. Try drinking a small glass every hour during the day.

Wash the affected areas carefully with a pH-balanced soap.

You can also try my 'kitchen cupboard treatment', a healing face mask:

2 tsp honey
¼ tsp fine sea salt
1 tsp turmeric

Mix into a thick paste and apply to spots overnight. Once spots have cleared, this makes a good preventative face-pack when applied once a month.

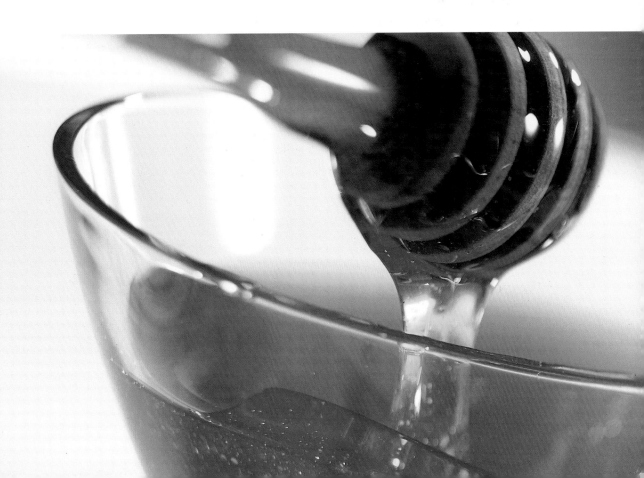

Acne Rosacea

This skin condition is often experienced in middle age, and is characterized by a flushed red face due to a weakness of the capillaries. Despite its name, it is a separate disorder from acne (see above) and does not have the characteristic pustules.

Acne rosacea is a condition of highly sensitive skin caused by an internal weakness or stress. It is linked to your environment (it is more common in colder countries) and also to the thickness of your epidermis, which is determined genetically. It is often accompanied by dryness or irritation around the chin, cheeks, nose and forehead, and is triggered in the highly sensitive mucous membranes of the nose, throat and sinuses in response to extremes of temperature, spicy foods, emotional distress, alcohol or hay fever. Attacks in response to the monthly hormone cycle are common.

Long term, acne rosacea leads to enlarged and broken blood vessels which are visible just under the skin. This is unfortunate because this can make you look like a drinker, even if you don't drink very much.

Treating Acne Rosacea

Unfortunately there is no medical cure. Instead, you need to learn to live with the condition and understand why your skin in reacting in this way to try and extend the period between attacks.

Ensure you are eating a sensible diet and drinking plenty of water.

The capillary networks can be strengthened by eating foods rich in vitamin E.

When the digestive tract and respiratory tract are clear, there is less likelihood of an attack.

Gargle with hot water, dissolving a quarter teaspoon of salt into a cup of hot water.

Polishing with a dab of pure castor oil and the lightest touch is advisable with acne rosacea. Dab the oil off with a three-ply tissue.

Cut out chocolate, coffee, orange juice, spices and alcohol (which can lead to the swollen red nose typical of the condition).

Take a daily vitamin B tablet.

Always use sunblock and wear a hat with a wide brim when out in the sunshine.

Drink eight glasses of water every day. If you drink alcohol, drink a glass or two of water for every glass of alcohol consumed.

Gargle with warm salt water each morning to ensure the infection does not spread to other parts of the face via the throat.

Apply Bach Flower Rescue Cream to the affected area each day.

Moisturize with almond oil or a little Vaseline.

Try to avoid stress, and pamper yourself a couple of nights a week with a warm bath and some quiet time.

Mix up a stabilizing face mask once a week:

1 heaped tsp chick-pea flour (available from healthfood shops or large supermarkets)
1 tsp double cream
2 tsp water
pinch of salt

Mix into a thick consistency and leave on for 10 minutes before rinsing off with lukewarm water.

Micro-dermabrasion can also help strengthen the skin (see page 163).

Tea Tree: The Natural Antiseptic

Tea tree oil, which is extracted from the manuka tree, is a bit of a skin magician. It's a natural antiseptic which, unlike some antiseptics, dissolves infection without damaging the skin. It sterilizes on contact and can prevent reinfection for hours. If you choose a cream that contains tea tree, dab it on twice a day with a cotton bud. If you are using neat tea tree oil on your skin, do a tiny patch test first as it can occasionally cause irritation in some people. Diluting it in olive oil (10 drops of olive oil to 1 or 2 drops of tea tree) is a safer approach if you are in any doubt.

Bags Under the Eyes

Dark circles under the eyes are an indication of stagnant circulation and pigment build-up which may be caused by hormonal imbalances, lack of sleep and a bad diet. Massage around the eyes towards the ears, with your ring fingers, to encourage the circulation to flow and reduce the severity of unsightly circles. Start where the eyebrow meets the bridge of the nose, applying deeper pressure at this point for a few seconds, then gently glide your finger just under the eyebrow, along the upper ridge of the eye socket, following through under each eye, twice daily.

Blackheads

When you have blackheads, you might imagine that they're caused by your pore becoming clogged by dirt. In fact, your pore is clogged, but with sebum, the body's own lubricant which is oxidized by the air and coloured with the skin's own pigment, melanin.

It's hugely tempting, but do *not* squeeze your blackheads. The skin is very vulnerable and the pressure required to loosen the blackhead can permanently damage your pores, bruise your skin, and cause further infection.

Treatments

The good news is that you can coax them out. The best approach is to create a home sauna with a basin of hot water. Pop a blanket over your head and tilt your head over the clouds of steam dissipating from the surface. Add a few drops of sage or aloe vera oil to the water to enhance the process. The heat will help to loosen blockages and encourage them to the surface where they are likely to pop out when washing.

Kaolin masks are another good approach. These are made from chalk, which absorbs the oil at the core of the blackheads.

Some people swear by blackhead papers. These strips are activated into a strong glue when in contact with water. Applied wet to your nose, chin, forehead or cheek, as the glue dries it bonds with the clogged sebum. Then, when you remove the strip, the sebum pops out too. These are a relatively expensive item, but can be extremely effective when carefully applied to smooth, acne-free skin once a month. They can lead to some reddening of

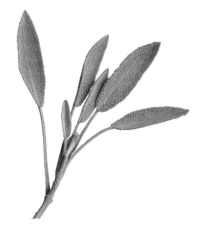

the skin, so you might want to use them at night before you go to sleep. The packets usually contain six or eight large strips, which you would use up very quickly. My advice is to cut each strip into smaller pieces which more accurately target the areas you want to treat. This can make peeling off the backing paper more difficult, but will save you money.

Eczema

This can be a very upsetting allergic condition. Skin becomes excessively dry and itchy in patches, and develops a rash that often weeps. Since the 1980s the number of children with the complaint has risen from one in eight to one in five. Two per cent of adults are also affected. It can be caused by an allergic reaction to a wide number of sensitizers including perfumes, houseplants, wool, stress, food additives and allergies, and the chemicals in make-up, shampoos, washing powder and body products.

Treatments

If you have an outbreak, try and work out what you have recently done that is different from your normal routine. Pay particular attention to your diet, and avoid the most common food allergens: eggs, peanuts, milk, fish, soy and wheat. Reintroduce them one by one, after two weeks' abstinence, and watch closely for flare-ups.

Taking a daily supplement of evening primrose oil for three months or more can reduce the symptoms of eczema. It's thought that the active ingredient in evening primrose oil, gamma-linolenic acid (GLA), can help reduce skin roughness.

Clinical studies have shown that the plant *Mahonia aquifolium* can be used both topically (on the outside) and internally to improve eczema. Traditionally it is used to treat fever, diarrhoea and rheumatic problems. The plant is rich in alkaloids which can help ease skin conditions. Order cream, bath oil or herbal extract from Jackson Ltd (see Resources chapter).

Drink plenty of water and try to avoid long-term use of steroid creams, which can cause the skin to thin, although they can be very useful periodically. Only use under your doctor's guidance.

It's very important to keep skin prone to eczema well moisturized to prevent itching. Apply almond oil liberally or choose an emollient cream such as aqueous cream, available from pharmacies, which contains none of the ingredients that can irritate sensitive skin. Generally ointments are best for very dry skin, and creams and lotions for 'wet' eczema.

Soak affected areas in Dead Sea salt baths. I believe passionately in these. The very high concentrations of minerals in the salts boost the skin's excretory function by dissolving the dehydrated dead cells which accumulate on the surface, particularly when the skin is overly dry and flaky.

Make up my kitchen cupboard treatment designed to calm inflamed skin:

2 tsp chickpea flour
2 tsp almond oil
¼ tsp salt

Apply to the affected area and leave for 10 minutes. Wash off with copious amounts of luke-warm water, and do not rub the skin. Pat dry very carefully.

In 2001, Marks & Spencer launched a range of clothing that aims to relieve some of the irritating symptoms of eczema. Designed with the help of eczema specialists from Great Ormond Street Children's Hospital, the 'Sensitive Skin' range is made of special fabrics that help prevent itching. The fabric contains *chitin*, a substance derived from the shells of Queen crabs that eases itching.

Wear cotton clothing next to the skin to keep the body cool. You should also avoid wool mixtures. Using non-biological washing powder, and avoiding fabric softener, can also help.

Liver Spots

These so-called 'age spots' have nothing whatsoever to do with the liver. They are actually sun spots, a form of large freckle that develops as a cumulative response to years of exposure to ultraviolet light, appearing years later following pigmentation changes deep within the skin. They often develop on the hands, and can also appear because of a deficiency of vitamin B-complex.

Treatment

Taking a daily vitamin B pill and using a high-factor sunblock on your hands can help prevent more from appearing, and reduce those you already have.

Moles

These are small raised clusters of skin pigment which often develop beneath the skin during adolescence. They are usually harmless, but if you notice a mole changing shape or becoming inflamed, or find an unusually shaped one, consult your doctor as this can be an indication of skin cancer.

Moles are usually trouble free, but irritations can result if they include a hair follicle which can become inflamed.

Treatments

If you are troubled by the way they look, moles can be removed by laser without leaving a scar.

Never pluck, wax or use depilatory cream to remove hairs from moles. Most moles remain harmless, but there is the risk that some can become cancerous – and disturbing them mechanically or chemically can exacerbate this.

The best way to deal with a hair emerging from a mole is to carefully snip it off where it is growing. You will need to do this once a week, so if the mole is in a prominent position and is affecting your confidence, consider having surgery to remove the entire mole along with the hair follicles within it. This can be done under local anaesthetic as an outpatient procedure, and modern techniques should not lead to scarring. Talk to your doctor first or seek private treatment.

Psoriasis

Sometimes confused with eczema, this is a genetic condition which can be triggered by diet, stress and illness. It is characterized by raised patches of pink and flaky skin which turn silver and drop off. New cells are produced at about 10 times normal speed, and this excessive growth leads to the constant shedding of large clumps.

Treatments

If you are suffering severely, your doctor can prescribe cortico-steroids. For less severe cases, Dead Sea mud salts can be added to the bath, and Dead Sea mud applied as a treatment. Coal tar soaps or Polytar shampoo can be helpful, as these help to regulate cell turnover. Taking a supplement of cod liver oil, which is rich in vitamin A, is useful for the same reason. Avoid coffee, citrus fruits and dairy products, and wear cool, loose clothing so your skin does not sweat.

Skin Tags

These are curious little outcroppings of skin that sometimes occur in middle age as a response to hormone changes. They are often seen on the neck or eyelids.

Treatments

Skin tags can be treated with high-current electrolysis. Alternatively, take a fine hair, loop into a knot, apply over the skin tag and tighten. Trim off the excess hair and, within a week or two, the skin tag will harmlessly drop off.

Warts

Take warts seriously. They are caused by an infectious virus which can cross-infect other parts of your body, entering into the skin through any cut or tiny fissure. They commonly occur on the feet, face, hands and knees. The characteristic hard lump is caused by the abnormal growth of skin cells.

Treatments

Ask your chemist for a homoeopathic or chemical remedy, and always wash your hands after you've touched the wart. Warts can also be removed by laser or cauterization. Ask your doctor.

how sunshine affects your skin

Our skin colour is inherited from our parents and controlled by a set of genes that dictate the amount of melanin within our skin. Melanin is produced by melanocytes, which send the pigment grains towards the surface, and their production is increased in the presence of ultraviolet rays.

The system is rather like those light-sensitive seventies sunglasses that automatically darkened when you went outside. It exists to protect the deeper layers of living skin cells from being burned. That explains why we get a suntan when we are exposed to sunlight. A suntan is the body's protective mechanism.

The skin of all races contains approximately the same number of melanocytes, but lighter-skinned people have a chemical in the skin which breaks down the melanin more quickly. Remember, if you find it difficult to get a tan that's because your skin is working particularly efficiently.

Your skin needs *some* sunshine. Too little exposure can be damaging, while too much sun thickens the epidermis and makes the skin leathery, lined and tough. Even if you don't burn, over-exposure to sunlight causes the skin to lose elasticity as the deep rays penetrate the skin all the way down to the dermis, leading to wrinkles which emerge years later. The sun is the cause of most wrinkles. Dry skin often results from sun-worshipping. Extreme exposure causes the development of melanoma (skin cancer).

However, hiding away in the dark is no solution. Some UV light is actually essential, and there is evidence that sensible amounts actually reduce the risk of other forms of cancer. Hormone levels, calcium absorption from the gut (which helps keep teeth and bones healthy and strong) and vitamin D-production are all controlled by sunlight. The danger lurks not in sunlight, but in sun*burn*.

As with so many things, the watchword here is *balance*. A light sun-kissed glow is all you need to feel and look wonderful. If turning mahogany is your ambition, look to a sunless tanning lotion instead. The days of the dreaded orange look have long passed and no one need know that your tan has come out of a bottle.

In the UK, around 130 times the amount of UV radiation reaches the skin at noon in the summer compared to the winter. In hot countries the locals stay in the shade between 11 a.m. and 3 p.m., but if you must go out a sunscreen is vital, whatever your skin type. Most fair skins can tolerate 15 minutes of sunshine before the skin starts to turn pink as it burns in the absence of sufficient melanin to protect it. The sun protection factor found on sunscreen lotions increases the amount of time you can spend in the sun by the number shown. A protection factor of 3 means that a fair-skinned person can stay in the sun for 45 minutes before burning. Bear in mind that sunscreens can easily be rubbed off, so it's a good idea to top them up every hour, whatever your skin type or the protection factor you have chosen.

Sunscreens work in two ways. They can contain either micro-reflective particles that act like a million tiny mirrors reflecting the damaging rays away from the skin, or chemicals that mop up the UV rays, a bit like melanin itself.

Always use a sunscreen, and supplement with a diet rich in vitamins E and C and beta-carotene to boost your natural resistance. These also help inhibit the development of cancer-causing compounds produced in the skin by exposure to excessive sunlight.

Safe Sun Care for Skin

Cover up when outside.

Always use a sun protection cream, or a face cream that includes it, even in mid-winter. UV rays can still cause damage even on a cold day.

Use a sunless bronzer to create a sun-kissed look.

Rather than sun-worshipping, spend your time outside being active.

Remember that the sun's rays are intensified by altitude and magnified by sun or snow. Use a higher protection factor in these conditions.

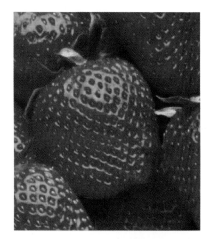

Take an evening primrose capsule every day to protect against skin damage caused by the sun, and to enhance the skin's health and suppleness.

Eat foods rich in antioxidants, to help the skin cope with the onslaught of UV rays: oranges, carrots, strawberries, raspberries, raisins, fresh cherries, sunflower seeds, fresh tomatoes, garlic, green salad, spinach, lime juice, and wheat germ.

If you are seeking a tan here's a three-point guide to achieving a golden glow:

1. Never sunbathe between 12 noon and 2.30 p.m., the time when the sun's rays are most damaging.
2. When you've spent a day in the sun, make sure you apply after-sun lotion to help prevent the skin drying out and leading to excess wrinkles.
3. Continue to cleanse, polish and moisturize your skin, which will prolong your tan and ultimately cut down the time you need to devote to tanning.

Home-made Sunscreen

You can make your own simple sunscreen, but if you intend to spend more than 30 minutes outside, supplement it with a clearly marked shop-bought sun protection factor cream.

3 tsp freshly squeezed lemon juice

1 tblsp aloe vera gel

2 capsules vitamin E oil

½ tsp carrot oil

6 drops orange essential oil

3 tblsp boiling water

Mix ingredients together and decant into a dark bottle. Apply half a teaspoon to the face two or three times a day. The mix is best kept in the fridge in the dark and will stay fresh for about 10 days.

Benefits of Sunshine

Sunlight offers us numerous physical benefits: UV rays stimulate the body's calcium and phosphate balance, encourage calcium absorption from the gut, and keep bones and teeth strong.

Disadvantages of Sunshine

Too much sunshine not only burns the skin but is the cause of premature ageing and can lead to melanoma (skin cancer).

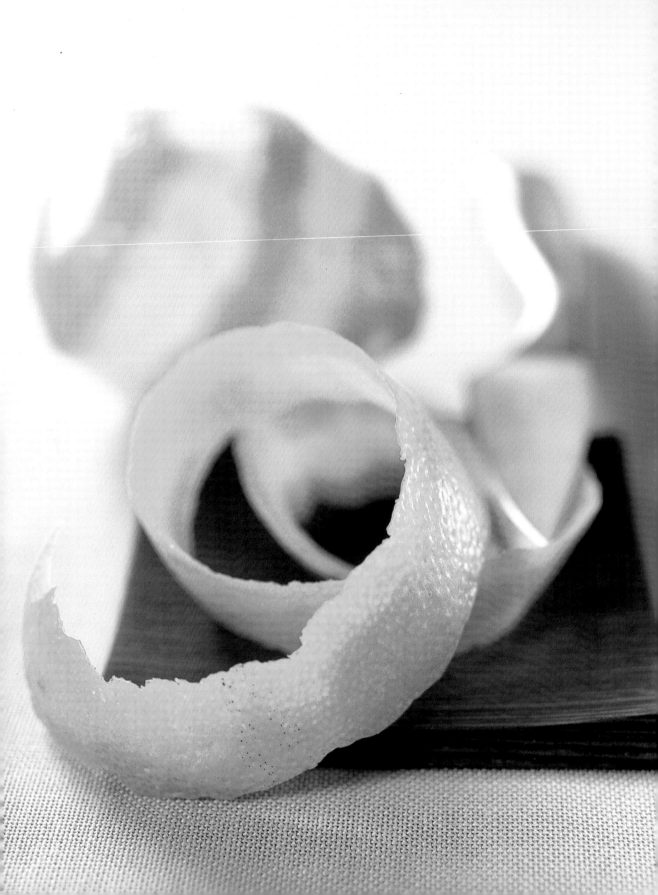

home-made cosmetics

Your kitchen cupboard is a source of natural ingredients, many of which are well-respected for their skin-care properties. The more unusual ingredients can be found in healthfood shops or Asian supermarkets.

Kitchen Cupboard Pharmacopoeia

Almonds	Exfoliate, soften, smooth and are a source of vitamin E
Apple cider vinegar	Similar pH to the skin's surface
Banana	Soothes sensitive skin and moisturizes
Cucumber	Soothes and tightens skin
Egg white	Tightens skin
Egg yolk	Moisturizes skin
Evening primrose oil	Moisturizes skin
Frankincense oil	Believed to aid with skin regeneration
Gram (chickpea) flour	Nourishes and cleanses the skin
Grapefruit juice	Tightens skin and is a natural antiseptic
Lemon peel	Tightens, lightens and is a natural antiseptic
Milk	Exfoliates, moisturizes and tightens skin
Mint	Tightens and refreshes the skin
Oatmeal	Exfoliates, soothes and is a source of vitamin E
Olive oil	Soothes and softens skin
Parsley	Tightens skin and has antiseptic properties
Rose water	A natural antiseptic that tightens and helps with skin regeneration
Sugar	An exfoliator that also tightens and is a natural antiseptic
Yoghurt	Exfoliates, soothes, moisturizes and tightens skin

recipes

Protein Exfoliator

Mix 1 teaspoon milk with 1 teaspoon finely ground almonds. The almonds have a light abrasiveness to them, but because they contain oil they will exfoliate without irritating the skin.

Coconut Oil and Honey Exfoliator

This is the lightest natural exfoliant. Mix up 1 teaspoon of each, polish, then wash with water.

Coffee Bean Cleanser

Grind a few fresh coffee beans and mix with 1 drop of almond oil to make a sweet-smelling cleanser.

Steaming Infusion for Oily Skin

A steam facial helps cleanse oily skin and unblock pores. Pour boiling water in a basin into which you have added 2 drops per litre of lavender, lemon or sandalwood essential oil, and a bunch of chopped mint or parsley. Cover your head with a towel and let the steam play over the surface of your skin for no longer than 10 minutes. Finish by splashing with cool water to close the pores. Avoid if you have acne or are prone to broken capillaries.

Lavender Cleanser for Oily Skin

Melt 2 tablespoons grated beeswax (available from healthfood shops) in a *bain-marie* (bowl suspended over a saucepan of boiling water). Remove from the heat and stir in 1 tablespoon sweet almond oil, 3 drops lavender oil and 1 dessertspoon mineral water. Smooth into your skin and remove with a tissue.

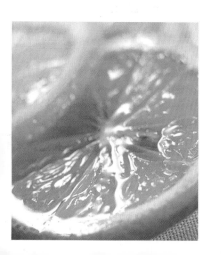

Zesty Spritzer for Oily Skin

Add 5 drops of freshly-squeezed lemon juice to a cup of hot water, stir in 3 drops of camomile essential oil and shake. Dab onto the skin after cleansing to refresh and help restore the skin's acid balance.

Healing Oil for Dry or Sensitive Skin

Pour 2 teaspoons pure wheat germ oil into a bottle. Add 2 teaspoons rose hip oil, 3 opened capsules of evening primrose oil and 2 drops geranium essential oil. Shake well. Dampen the face and neck slightly, and apply a little oil with your fingers, letting it be absorbed into the skin for about a quarter of an hour before applying make-up.

Moisturizer for Different Skin Types

Melt 1 tablespoon beeswax in a *bain-marie* (bowl suspended over a saucepan of boiling water) and beat in 3 tablespoons vegetable oil (one or more of the following: olive, sweet almond, sunflower, evening primrose). Remove from the heat and add 1 tablespoon rose water. Continue to stir as the liquid cools. When lukewarm, stir in the contents of a vitamin E capsule and 3 drops of essential oil appropriate to your skin type:

For normal or dry skin Lavender, neroli, rose, camomile or elder flower

For oily skin Sandalwood, cedar wood or cardamom

Use within two weeks, longer if kept refrigerated.

Simple Moisturizer

A quick way to make up your own moisturizer is to put a dab of sesame or almond oil on your palm and add a drop of warm water. Rub briskly between your palms to emulsify the oil and water, and apply to your skin.

For Sensitive Skin: Gentle Honey Polisher

If your skin is very sensitive, mix 1 teaspoon honey with a few drops of boiling water to polish it and remove dead skin cells. Using small upward motions, gently rub the honey into your skin. Dead cells will stick to the honey. Wash off with plenty of warm water.

Oatmeal Polisher

This is one of the best and most simple of all home-made beauty products, and I swear by it. Mix 2 tablespoons finely ground oatmeal with 1 tablespoon almond oil. Stir into a sticky mix and use it to polish your face.

Facial Polisher for All Skin Types

Polishing is a mainstay of my approach to beauty care. Mix up your own gentle polisher: Add 1 dessertspoon finely ground almonds to 1 teaspoon finely ground oatmeal and 1 teaspoon gram flour. Add 1 dessertspoon almond oil, 2 teaspoons aloe vera juice and 4 drops tea tree oil. Pour in a small amount of boiling water to thin if necessary, and polish gently into the face, avoiding the delicate eye area.

An even simpler mix for dry skin: Mix together 2 tablespoons finely ground oatmeal with 1 tablespoon almond oil. Massage all over the body using your palms to produce the best results. The polisher will remove dead skin cells and moisturize the skin.

Gram Flour Firming Mask

Gram (chickpea) flour is a cosmetic staple in Indian households, and recipes using it offer an effective way to cleanse and nourish the skin. Mix 1 heaped teaspoons gram flour with 2 teaspoons water and half a teaspoon honey. Apply this creamy paste to your face and leave for 15 minutes.

To treat sensitive skin, add 1 teaspoon double cream.

Milk Exfoliating Cleanser

Milk is an excellent cleanser which gently dissolves away dead skin cells while not affecting the skin's natural pH. Add 1 drop of essential oil suitable for your type (see home-made soap recipe, page 46) to 1 dessertspoon of milk. Soak cotton wool in the mixture and wipe over the face before washing away with warm water. For dry skin, add a pinch of finely chopped fresh parsley. For oily, add a pinch of chopped mint.

Natural Facial Peel

Use sparingly to exfoliate by dissolving the natural glue that binds dead skin cells together. Take 1 teaspoon of your most gentle face cream and mix into it 1 teaspoon of freshly squeezed pineapple. Massage around the nose and cheeks, avoiding the eye area. Leave for a couple of minutes and splash away. Skin may tingle as the weak alpha-hydroxyl acid solution is working.

Alternatively, gently rub a slice of apple over the skin to help lift loose cells. Wash with warm water afterwards.

Humble Potato Mask

Grate a potato and apply the raw pulp all over your face. The potassium it contains is particularly good for sunburn. Alternatively, slice discs of potato and apply around the nose and over closed eyelids for an invigorating tonic.

Cucumber Lifting Face Pack

This is the simplest way to give yourself an instant face-lift. Chop six inches of cucumber into thick slices and liquidize in a blender into a smooth pulp. Sit back and gently massage into your face, leaving it covered in a thick layer. Leave for no longer than 30 minutes before rinsing with warm water and patting until dry. Follow with moisturizer to seal in a thin layer of moisture.

Delicious Banana and Honey Moisturizing and Exfoliating Mask

This recipe smells a treat as well as producing great results for your skin. Simply mash half a banana and add 2 tablespoons natural bio yoghurt and 1 tablespoon honey. Mix together to form a paste. Use immediately and leave on no longer than 30 minutes. Dab off with a soft cotton cloth or three-ply tissue, and rinse with plenty of warm water.

Fruit Mask

Use a blender to create a thick cream out of any combination of pineapple, strawberries and kiwi fruit, and stir in a small amount of milk powder to absorb the watery part. Gently cover your face in a thin layer of almond oil and apply the fruit mask. Leave on for 15 minutes. The fruit acids will be absorbed into the oil (applying them directly is too acidic for the skin).

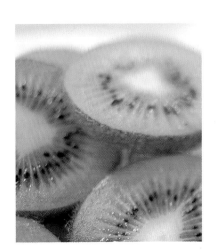

Home-made Soap

You can create your own custom soap by grating a bar of soap into flakes and placing in a glass bowl over a saucepan of boiling water. Add 1 cup of boiling water and 8 drops of essential oil:

For normal skin	geranium, rose or coconut
Dry skin	elder flower or camomile
Sensitive skin	frankincense
Oily skin	rosemary or lemon

If you wish to create an exfoliating soap, add 2 teaspoons ground oatmeal or rice flour. For a moisturizing soap, add 1 teaspoon honey.

Choose a suitable mould and line with parchment, spoon the mixture in and leave overnight in the fridge. Store in a cool place.

Lip Plumper

Lips have no sebaceous glands of their own, and need the added lubrication of balm throughout the year. One of the most effective ways to plump up your lips is to smear a drop of castor oil on them. Alternatively, make your own lip conditioner by mixing together half a teaspoon Aloe Vera gel with a pea-sized drop of vitamin E cream and 6 drops rose oil. Rub into your lip lines every day.

Honey Lip Salve

Melt 1 tablespoon beeswax in a *bain-marie* (bowl suspended over a saucepan of boiling water) and remove from the heat. Stir in 2 tablespoons sweet-almond oil and 1 teaspoon honey. Decant and use within six weeks.

Frown Line Relaxer

Often we are left with deep furrows between our eyebrows after habitual patterns of stress and concentration. Try this recipe to help relax the frown. Pour one-eighth cup rose water in a bowl and add 1 drop neroli oil. Stir in 1 ounce ground almonds and the contents of one vitamin E capsule. Dip a cotton wool pad into the mixture and lay it over your frown lines for about 45 minutes while lying down.

Refreshing Eye Treatment

Every morning, revitalize your eyes by splashing with water. Better still is to boil up a saline and water solution, using 1 pint of water and 1 teaspoon table salt boiled together. Cool and store in the fridge. Bathe your eyes with this every morning.

Gentle Eye Gel

The skin around the eyes is particularly delicate. Make your own light eye gel by mixing a dessertspoon of aloe vera gel with the contents of one capsule of vitamin E oil and 8 drops evening primrose oil. Keep in the fridge and apply daily.

Eye Mask

Grate a chunk of cucumber and strain off 1 teaspoon of the juice. Stir into 1 tablespoon of powdered milk to make a thick paste. Close the eyes and apply to upper and lower lids. Leave for 10 minutes, then wipe off gently with a moist tissue.

Elixirs of Youth

Natural skin-care ingredients to help prevent or disguise premature ageing include:

Antioxidants	Oatmeal, carrot oil, wheatgerm oil, ground almonds
Soothers	Yoghurt, olive oil
Moisturizers	Jojoba oil, apricot kernel oil, sweet almond oil, evening primrose oil
Skin tighteners	Honey, egg whites, cucumber, lemon juice
Skin-cell regenerators	Rose water, neroli oil, frankincense oil

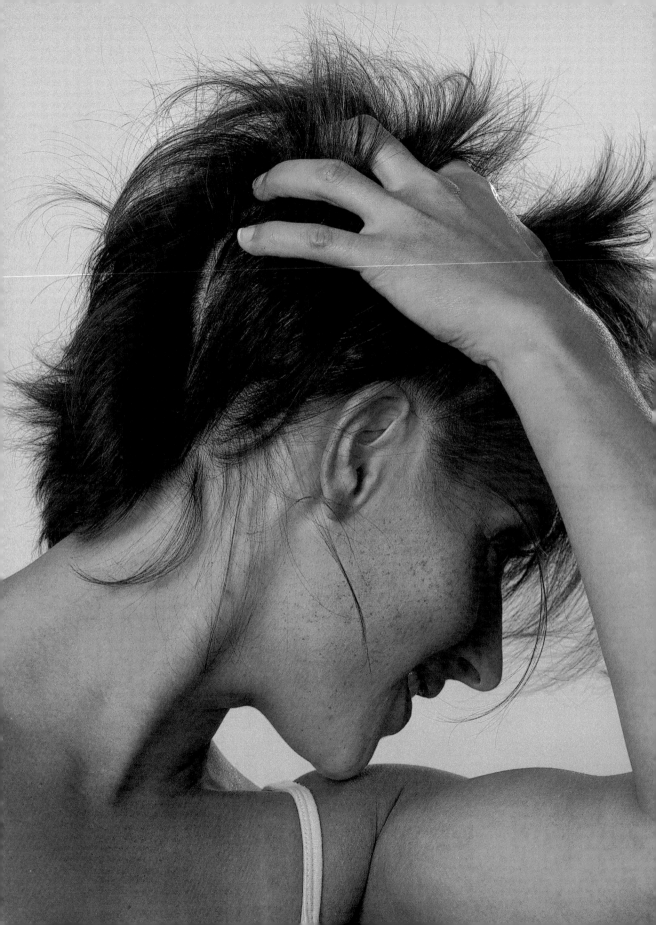

your hair

'Hair is like ivory, it's both dead and delicate.' I love this saying. Hair is also like the rings of a tree. It can't tell you your age, but you can read your history in it. The creation of hair is fed by the blood supply, and all aspects of our nutrition and lifestyle is minutely reflected in it.

If you want luscious, shiny, flattering locks, the best way to get them is to eat a balanced, nutrient-rich diet. That's the prevention-rather-than-cure approach. You only need to spend money on potions and unguents if you've neglected to create healthy-looking hair, or failed to treat it properly by choosing products that are too harsh, getting yourself into a vicious cycle of greasy/dry. Mild shampoos are better than harsh ones, gentle brushes and combs preferable to harsh metal versions.

Hair care is a multi-million pound industry because hair is all about sensuality. In other animals it may have additional uses – to protect, to warm, to camouflage – but in humans our hair is tied up with sexual reproduction. Healthy, glossy, radiant hair is an advertisement for our fecundity. The way we style it is a sign of the personality we wish to project. Given that first impressions are formed within three seconds of meeting someone, you owe it to yourself to make yours as healthy and expressive as you are.

How to Frame Your Face

If you are in any doubt about how important your hair is to your confidence and the image you project, just cast your mind back to your last 'bad hair day' and how self-conscious it made you feel. A recent study into self-image found that 'bad hair awareness' – hair that sticks out, needs cutting, is flyaway, badly cut, bushy, greasy, frizzy, damaged or wild – negatively influences self-esteem, brings out social insecurities and causes people to focus on the worst aspects of themselves.

You produce an average of seven miles of hair a year, and it needs constant care if it is to stay looking lustrous for the years that each strand will stay on your head.

We face an onslaught of anti-hair agents in modern life: pollution, excessive styling, sunbathing, hair dryers, stress, lack of exercise and countless chemicals that are supposedly 'enhancing' our hair.

So take your hair seriously and don't feel guilty about spending some time caring for it. Time was when any greying British woman over the age of 60 automatically conformed, opting for a 'poodle perm' – short tight curls worn like a helmet, which seemed to spell out the dreadful letters OAP. Thankfully, mature women now have the option of choosing from a far wider range of styles.

To make the most of yourself, you need to consider your face shape and your age as well as the condition, colour and texture of your hair in order to make an informed decision about how best to wear it to enhance your appearance.

Hair Styles to Adapt to Face Shape

In the same way that you dress your body to enhance your body shape – compensating for narrow shoulders with subtle shoulder pads, or playing down big hips by wearing dark colours while drawing attention upwards with a colourful print – so too your hair can be used to dress up your natural face shape.

Cut and coloured correctly, your hairstyle can flatter your facial structure and effectively draw attention away from features such as a large nose or pointed chin that you may prefer to disguise.

Round Face

Choose a style that adds volume to the top of your head, rather than the sides, and opt for a soft (rather than a sharply cut) style. It's best to avoid long hair or a chin-length bob, which will emphasize the moon-like quality of your face. Your best choice is a structured cut with the use of mousse or spray to prevent the extra height you've gained from flopping over as the day goes on. Avoid a heavy blunt fringe, which will make your face appear wider – however, a light feathered fringe will help break up the overall circularity of your face. Bringing hair forward onto the cheeks will help reduce width. Adding a bit of asymmetrical focus, such as a side parting or hair that is swept back on one side only, helps to vary the rhythm of your face's natural outline.

Long Face

Try to add volume and energy to the hair either side of your face, while downplaying its height. Aim for some structured or fluffy fullness around the cheekbones and ears, rather than the cheeks, so your face does not appear to 'puddle' towards the jawline. Central partings should be avoided, particularly if your hair is straight, as they draw attention to the face's narrowness. Instead, choose a strong side parting which helps to offset the length of your face by introducing some asymmetry and appearing to widen the cheekbones.

Angular Diamond-shaped Face

Consider a classic rounded bob which falls to the chin – this will emphasize the attractive angularity of your face, while rounding out your chin. You can also afford a heavy fringe to add width across your forehead, but avoid adding volume at the cheekbones.

Heart-shaped Face

To downplay a pointed chin, you want to avoid making your face appear to taper. A chin-length bob is a very good choice, as are curls that draw the eye to the chin area, both of which will add fullness at chin level. Emphasize softness and curves, and avoid a sharp angled cut. You can also use an off-centre parting to soften and narrow your wider forehead.

Square Face or Prominent Jaw

Go for a super-feminine, feathered cut that allows wisps of hair to fall onto the face at chin level, masking the angularity of your features. Keep your hair long enough to soften your chin line. A bob or a super-long, super-straight style are very bad ideas, as both make the face's structure overly prominent. But you can get away with a short geometric cut that adds height to create fullness if you want to look strong and make an impact.

Oval Face

This symmetrical face shape gives you lots of latitude in how you wear your hair, but you should avoid a long fringe, which will throw off the balance of the face. More than any other face shape, you can afford to wear your hair back from your face; a chignon is wonderfully flattering, and even a simple ponytail looks good on your underlying even bone structure.

How to Disguise Specific Features

Large Nose

First, always remember that your nose feels larger to you than to anyone else. If you are conscious of it, you will tend to focus on it when you look in the mirror, to the exclusion of the rest of your face, but other people will see your face in context. Choose a hairstyle that brings your hair forward over your cheeks and builds up volume towards the crown and back of your head. This will help draw attention away from your nose.

Long Neck

A long neck is a boon, unless you over-emphasize it, so it's best to stick with longer styles that will show off your hair rather than risk appearing out of balance with a short style. Opting for a style that is wider and fuller at the back, rather than a style that tapers to a point, is also preferable.

Short Neck

Avoid long styles, which will minimize further the gap between your chin and shoulders. A short style, perhaps even cut up the neck, will elongate your neck line.

Low Forehead

You want to give the illusion that your forehead is higher than it really is, so the key is to mask the hair line. A short, feathered fringe can achieve this when coupled with a style adding height to the top of your head.

High Forehead

Opt for a style that incorporates a fringe, and if you have long hair that you tie back, pull out of a few longer tendrils to softly flatter the face and draw attention downwards.

Protruding Ears

Obscure them with a cut that is full enough to cover the front and back of your ears. If you have fine hair and are extremely conscious about having slightly larger ears, you might want to consider a soft perm that will allow your ears to disappear in some softly sculpted curls.

hair types

Your hair is made up of 3 per cent moisture and 97 per cent dead protein. Not a very appealing statistic, so it's reassuring how lustrous and beautiful this unpromising raw material can appear, despite the fact that most hairs will stay attached to your head for between three and seven years. The average head has over 100,000 hairs which grow at the rate of half an inch a month and shed at the rate of 50 to 100 a day. If your hair is 12 inches in length, you are losing up to 100 feet of hair a day, so you can expect your hairbrush to need regular unpicking – it doesn't necessarily mean you have a hair-loss problem. You can lose half your hair before it noticeably thins.

Problems that arise with hair function as a signpost to your internal health. What many people do not realize is that healthy hair is dependent on a healthy *scalp*. Poor circulation can often contribute to a variety of hair problems. The tens of thousands of follicles crammed into this covering of skin need to be sufficiently fed. When blood is not flowing freely this can lead to stagnant circulation, resulting in toxic build-up.

Age, health, diet, hormones, climate and seasonal changes are all factors that affect hair growth and health. Stress and anxiety are also significant factors, because they cause blood to be diverted to other parts of the body, resulting in reduced oxygen supply to the scalp which means hair eventually looks less healthy.

Regular head massages for the stressed-out are therefore rather useful, as they help to reactivate blood flow (see pages 66 and 94).

caring for different hair conditions
Dry Hair

This can be caused by the under-activity of sebaceous glands in the scalp, poor circulation or because of a deficiency of zinc or fatty acids in the body. Split ends are caused when a protein called *keratin* in the hair is reduced. Keratin helps the hair to lock up moisture, so the result of its absence is dry, brittle hair prone to snapping.

Choose a shampoo with the active cleansing ingredient *laureth sulphate*, recommended for dry hair because of its inherent conditioning properties (its cousin, *lauryl sulphate*, is too harsh for dry hair and has been linked to eczema).

Using 1 teaspoon coconut oil on the hair once a week will help it look wonderfully glossy. Massage into your hands and stroke through the hair, then leave overnight. This is a super greasy oil, so use sparingly and wash your hair thoroughly the following morning.

If you want to use a shop-bought conditioner, apply to the mid-lengths of the hair and the ends, where the hair has been exposed to the elements longest. If your hair is very dry, apply 1 tablespoon live yoghurt once a week after washing, leave for a minute, then rinse.

If you suffer from split ends, have your hair cut every eight weeks. All you need to remove is the bottom half-inch. If you are growing your hair you'll still be growing double what you are cutting off.

Choose a conditioner with *hydrolysed proteins* in it. These penetrate and temporarily strengthen the hair shaft, and can be a good way to prevent split ends, commonly associated with over-dry hair.

Using a hair dryer while the hair is any wetter than half-dry will cause too much moisture to be sucked out of it. Use a dryer to 'finish off' drying your hair, and only on a cooler setting. Your hair will then be much less prone to frizz. Use alcohol-free gels to avoid drying out the hair.

Greasy Hair

If your hair is producing too much sebum (natural oil), your hair may appear limp and greasy. The over-activity of oil-producing glands is influenced by hormones and heredity, so you can't do much to change the cause, although you can minimize the effects.

Shampoos commonly contain one of two active ingredients: *lauryl sulphate* and *laureth sulphate*, both of which clean without leaving a residue, as soap does. *Lauryl sulphate* is the active ingredient to look for if your hair is naturally oily, as it cleans well but does not condition – but bear in mind it has been linked to eczema.

It can be hard to find shampoos specifically designed for oily hair. Choose one that says 'deep cleansing' or 'for fine, limp hair' if you are stuck. You don't need a protein-rich shampoo, as this will make your hair feel heavier and limper still.

People with oily hair should condition less. Once a week is usually sufficient, and concentrate on the ends only. Disperse the scalp's natural oils through the hair every day by brushing upside-down for 50 strokes.

If you fear your hair is greasy or limp because of a build-up of hair treatment products, use a clarifying shampoo, such as Neutrogena, once a week to remove residue.

Curly Hair

Curly hair curls because the hair shaft is oval rather than round, which leads the hair shaft to twist slightly as it emerges from the scalp. This is a genetic inheritance, so if you want straight hair your best choice is a relaxant perm.

Curly hair is prone to being dry, so use a deep conditioner once a week, and a moisturizer or gloss on the ends to give sheen.

Enjoy your naturally curly hair – most people with straight hair would die for some natural curl.

Permed or Chemically-treated Hair

Chemically treating your hair can give you the lift you require, offering curls where you had dead straight locks, straightening out frizzy hair, or giving you a colour that increases your confidence. The downside is that your hair is now more fragile and needs extra care to help it hang on to moisture.

Avoid over-heating hair, either with water or with the heat of the hairdryer, and let it dry naturally if you can.

It's very important to use conditioner or hair-moisturizer if your hair is treated. The hair shaft has been damaged by the chemical process involved and is therefore less able to hold on to moisture. Using a good conditioner helps smooth out the hair cuticle and restore sheen. Instant leave-in conditioners are great for chemically-treated hair. A deep conditioning treatment used weekly will help restore shine and elasticity.

If you use a wash-in or semi-permanent hair colour, bear in mind that the weakened structure of chemically-treated hair

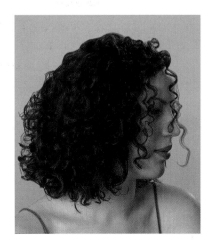

means that the colour is likely to be locked into the hair shaft for longer, rather than merely coating the exterior of each hair, so colour absorption will be more intense and the results are likely to last longer.

Look for 'quaternary ammonium' compounds on the ingredients label of your conditioner. These improve shine and improve manageability for dyed or permed hair.

hair disorders

Dandruff

Dandruff is an excess of dead skin cells that are not only embarrassing but also make hair look dull and lifeless, as they clog the oil glands that keep hair looking glossy and smooth.

Dandruff can be aggravated by a dry scalp, harsh shampoos, improper rinsing after using shampoo, poor diet, some medications and hot, spicy foods. One of the best over-the-counter remedies is Polytar Liquid shampoo.

Alternatively, take a vitamin E tablet daily and help to calm your scalp by mixing the yolk of one egg with half a teaspoon lemon juice and 2 drops camphor. Massage gently into the scalp and leave for 10 minutes before rinsing with copious lukewarm water (don't use hot water, you'll end up with scrambled egg in your hair!).

Dandruff is the result of a build-up of dead cells which occurs when the hair follicles do not receive enough nourishment. This also affects the shine and lustre of the hair. Regular scalp polishing can help remedy this. Apply the scalp polisher to a dry head of hair, starting at the forehead point of the hair line and working towards the back of the head, covering every inch of the scalp. Massage the scalp vigorously with the balls of the fingers. The moment water is applied, the scalp polisher becomes a shampoo. This method of scalp polishing will increase circulation to the scalp and strengthen the hair roots. Try to make this become a regular routine to avoid scalp problems.

Head Lice

It's not an urban myth designed to make you feel better, head lice really do like clean hair. If hair is greasy they climb as far as they can down the shaft to cleaner territory, even going without the life-giving blood (yours) that they need to survive. There is one vital watchword with lice: *speed*. Yours, not theirs. If you see a louse, you've got a problem you must deal with immediately. With more than a 10th of a million hairs on your head they've got plenty of places to hide, and as soon as you find one, see an egg case (nit) stuck to a hair, or feel an itching at the back of your neck where they like to hang out (it's warm and dark there), you've got a great deal more you haven't met yet. Unfortunately they are all extremely busy laying eggs and perpetuating the next generation. And even though it's easy to kill the fully-grown louse with special-ized lotion, the eggs come encased in a hard silvery shell which means some of them are likely to survive treatment – and the more that survive, the more that will hatch a few weeks later.

You can buy effective over-the-counter lotions which will kill lice and their eggs, but your hair will still contain the egg cases, which can be unsightly. These can be removed by a specialized fine-toothed metal comb (also available from the chemist) which will also remove the dead lice. Take hair in small sections and comb repeatedly, rinsing the metal comb after each stroke.

To help prevent reinfection, massage half a teaspoon tea tree oil once a month into the scalp of towel-dried hair, making sure you don't overlook the nape of your neck.

Greying Hair

This is a genetic condition. It occurs when insufficient melanin pigment is produced in the hair follicle to maintain its original colour, but it is sometimes linked to an iron deficiency, particularly in vegetarians. If your mother and grandmother went grey when they were young, you might find you have inherited a tendency to prema-ture greying.

Whatever the cause, I'm an advocate of tinting or colour-treating hair, as it's a simple short-cut back to confidence. I've been using colour for years. No one guesses because I've chosen a colour which is close to my natural colour and I am gradually lightening it as I get older to match the pigmentation changes of my skin. If your hair is brown, don't use henna as it colours the greying hairs red, making them all too obvious (see Colouring Your Hair, page 59).

Stress, anger, the menopause, thyroid problems, and a lack of copper, zinc or folic acid can sometimes lead hair to lose its colour.

Have a thyroid test to check yours is not under- or over-active. Choose a diet rich in nuts, minerals and protein. Increase your intake of vitamin E, an anti-ageing antioxidant found in almonds, avocados, brown rice, leafy greens, hazelnuts, oatmeal, peanut butter, sunflower seeds and wholemeal flower. B-complex vitamins are also useful, as they help to metabolize carbohydrates and proteins. They are found in a range of foods including whole grains, brewer's yeast and dairy products, or take a multi-vitamin.

Thinning Hair

As you grow older hair grows more slowly and thins due to the action of the thymus gland. Thirty per cent of women will notice some thinning of their hair by the age of 50, while 50 per cent of men will lose some hair by the age of 30. The difference is that women tend to lose hair from all over the scalp, while male hair loss is concentrated into particular zones, such as the crown or temples. This is known as 'male pattern balding'.

When we are stressed and as we age, the thymus gland produces less of the hormone thymolin, which leads to our follicles letting go of the hair they contain. Thinning hair is also exacerbated by poor diet, the over-use of a hairdryer, alcohol and smoking, all of which lead to decreased blood flow and reduced oxygen reaching the scalp. It can also be caused by the hormones in HRT, as well as being connected to a change in thyroid levels at the time of the menopause. A trip to the doctor is a good idea if you are concerned. You may be suffering from a medical condition, *alopecia* (hair loss) or *alopecia arebets* (bald patches).

The good news is that female hair loss is easier to treat than male hair loss. With hormone treatment and correct nutrition, women with genetic hair thinning can expect up to 40 per cent re-growth.

If you don't want to take a pharmacological approach, a weekly scalp massage (see below) can help reduce the symptoms.

Stick to healthy fresh foods, rather than processed alternatives, to give your follicles the nutrients they need to produce healthy hair: like a plant, the hair is governed by its living roots. Your hair needs eight essential amino acids to stay healthy. Eating millet is a great hair-booster as it contains seven of these acids as well as growth-promoting vitamin B. Use instead of rice or pasta, or add flakes of it to muesli.

colouring your hair

There is only one reason to colour your hair: to make you feel better about yourself. If you like your hair colour, be it dark brown or naturally greying, then leave it alone. Dying your hair with anything stronger than a wash-in/wash-out colour damages the hair shaft and will require more attention. That said, you can have a lot of fun giving yourself a temporary wash-in tint that lasts for several washes.

If you do want to colour-treat your hair more permanently, make sure you find a colour that complements your skin tone so that your hair looks naturally flattering, rather than out of place.

When applied correctly the right colour can give texture and volume to thin hair, add shine, depth and movement, brighten your face, make you look younger and enhance existing natural colour. Incorrectly applied it can give hair the texture of straw, jar with your natural colouring to age you, and look lifeless.

Older women should avoid slavishly trying to match hair tone to the colour you once had. Skin tones also lose pigment over time, and the contrast can appear too obvious.

Highlighting is a good way to begin to add more vibrancy to your hair, especially if the streaks are applied in several different shades. A couple of shades of blonde can give life to blonde hair. For dark hair, choose shades of red, dark honey or bronze, but if you are brunette avoid light blonde highlights – your hair will look unnatural and will clash with your eyebrows.

If you colour your hair at home, apply a smear of Vaseline around your hair line to prevent your skin from being coloured, and use rubber gloves to stop the colour getting under your nails.

Here is my guide to timeless hair colour:

Dark Brown or Black Hair/Blue, Green or Hazel Eyes/Light Skin

Because of your light skin and bright eyes you can go blonde if you want a real change of image, and soften your look considerably. If you want to enhance your natural colour, choose an auburn or copper. To add contrast, choose dark brown or chestnut brown highlights.

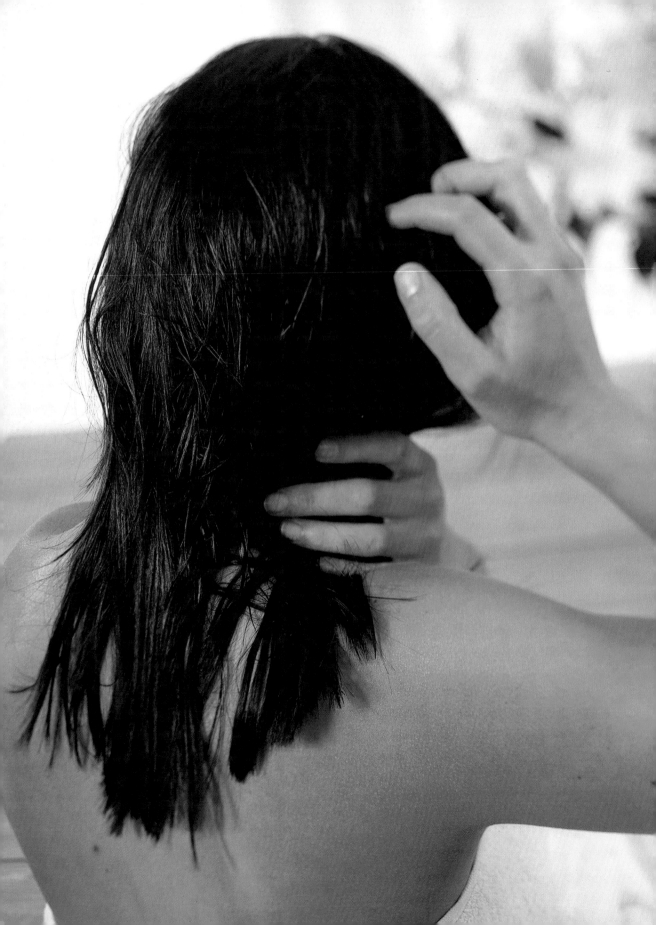

Dark Hair and Eyes/Medium or Olive Skin Tone

Try mahogany, chestnut or copper tones. Your natural colour will not lighten but will glow with a sheen of the new colour. If you want to lighten your hair a little, add subtle highlights in a colour just two shades lighter than your own.

Blonde Hair/Hazel, Brown or Green Eyes/Golden Skin Tone

Try adding golden, copper or honey shades to flatter your hair colouring. If you have green eyes, try using a brighter auburn or Titian red. If your eyes are darker, try darker auburn or copper.

Light to Medium Blonde or Brown/Hazel or Brown Eyes/Medium Skin Tone

Your colouring is muted. You will lighten your look if you choose several shades of blonde highlights, and look more vibrant if you select medium to deep shades of chestnut. Avoid using red – your delicate facial and eye colouring will appear washed out.

Medium to Light Blonde Hair/Blue, Green or Grey Eyes/Medium Skin Tone

Add medium-blonde shades to give richness and depth. Try strawberry or honey shades for a lighter look. If you have bright blue or green eyes, you can use a more potent copper or mahogany colour effectively.

home-made hair treatments and treats

A common beauty myth is that in order for a shampoo to clean your hair effectively you need to achieve that 'squeaky clean' feeling. This is bunkum. The squeaky-clean feeling is evidence that your hair has been stripped not only of the dirt you do want to remove, but also of all the necessary oils that your hair naturally produces to help it stay moist and healthy. 'Squeaky clean' has to be followed by conditioner, because if you don't put back a certain amount of greasy moisture into your hair, it will soon be a dry, brittle mess.

A light coating of natural oil produced from the hair follicle helps to give hair a natural shine, but the trouble with the modern approach to hair cleansing is that it upsets the natural balance of sebum produced by your hair follicles and your hair tends to over-compensate, becoming greasy more quickly and needing washing more often.

Vegetable-based shampoos and some of the more expensive shampoos available from your hair salon are a good investment, but don't expect them to lather. We expect a shampoo to lather to show that it is working, but a shampoo that offers that reassuringly thick white bubbly blanket is simply a shampoo that contains the sudsing phosphates you'd be better off avoiding.

To give your hair a special treat, make your own hair treatments using herbs sourced from your local healthfood shop. These should all be stored in the fridge between treatments, and used within seven days.

Kitchen Cupboard Shampoo

Mix 3 tablespoons of the relevant herb for your scalp type (see below) with a cup of water, bring to the boil and then simmer on a low flame until half the liquid has evaporated. Sieve and decant. Add 1 dessertspoon liquid olive soap (available from healthfood stores) and stir into an even paste.

Herb Types

Oily scalp	Bay leaf or rosemary
Sensitive scalp	Camomile
Dry scalp	Lavender

Wash your hair using 1 teaspoon of the shampoo. Rinse with plenty of water and pat hair dry. Massage scalp with 2 drops lavender (dry scalp) or rosemary (oily scalp) essential oils before leaving to dry.

Kitchen Cupboard Weekly Conditioner

Make a paste using 1 teaspoon of each of the following: neem, sandalwood, triphala and licorice powder. Mix with 2 tablespoons warm water. Apply to dry scalp and comb through with a wide-toothed comb. Leave on for half an hour, then rinse with warm water.

Mayonnaise massaged into the hair once a week and washed away with cool water is a great protein-rich treat for hair.

Kitchen Cupboard Scalp Polisher

Mix 1 dessertspoon yoghurt with 1 teaspoon olive oil and half a teaspoon lemon juice. Add 1 dessertspoon rice flour. Massage and gently polish the scalp. Rinse off thoroughly with warm water. This product treats the scalp, helps remove flaking skin, and conditions the hair roots for a healthy, well-nourished shine.

Kitchen Cupboard Natural Colour

Mix 3 tablespoons of the herb appropriate to your hair colour (see below) with a cup of water, bring to the boil and simmer until the liquid reduces by half. Sieve and decant. Apply after shampooing and leave on for 5 minutes, then rinse thoroughly and use the hair glosser below if required.

For dark brown hair	Ground walnuts
For blonde hair	Camomile flowers
For red hair	Henna paste or a pinch of saffron
For black hair	Sage

All hair types can get that sun-lightened look by pouring 1 teaspoon diluted lemon juice over the hair before going out in the sun (remember to condition later). Alternatively, draw strands of hair across a cut lemon to give a subtle highlight.

Avoid using strong peroxide on your hair in the search for instant blonde. If you've got any underlying red you're likely to become a carrot top, and trying to compensate with colour can turn your hair green.

Kitchen Cupboard Hair Glosser

Steep the juice of half a lemon in a cup of boiling water and rinse hair in this lemony-scented liquid after you've shampooed. Do not rinse out.

Peach-nut oil can be used to give a wonderful natural sheen to dry hair by dropping 3 or 4 drops into your palms, rubbing them together vigorously and brushing your hands lightly over your hair, concentrating on the lengths and ends.

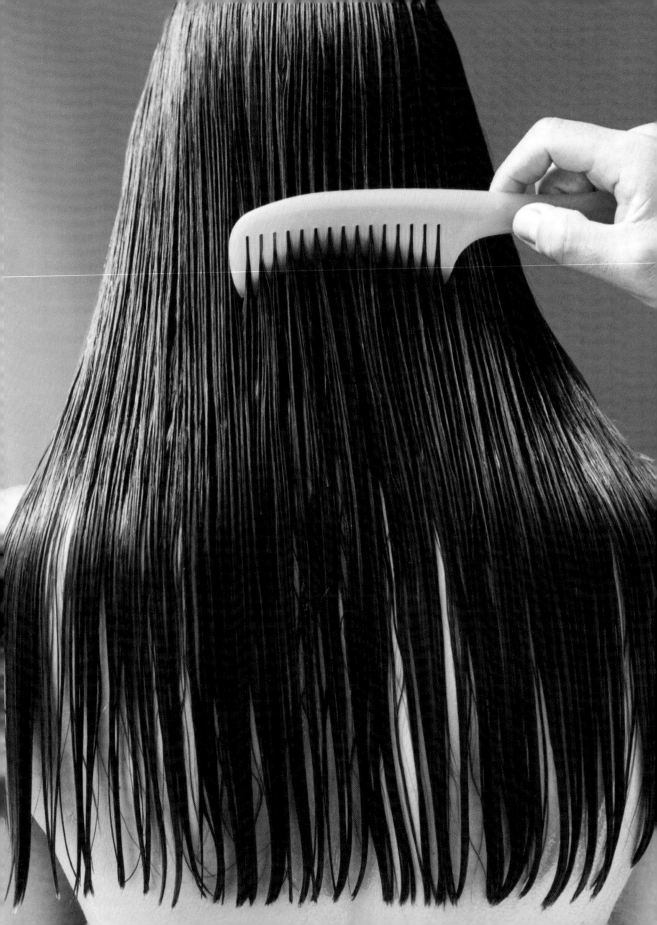

One reason conditioner makes hair shine is because it restores its acid/alkali balance. You can do the same by putting a dessertspoon of vinegar in the final rinse to make your hair shine.

Kitchen Cupboard Gel

Mix up gelatine and water to create a natural setting gel, increasing the proportion of gelatine to water for a firmer set. But bear in mind that gelatine is not suitable for strict vegetarians, who might prefer to use beer (the smell wears off after a few minutes!).

Kitchen Cupboard Intensive Hair Massage Oil

Only use this recipe if you have a dry or sensitive scalp or are suffering from dandruff. This is a good evening treatment once a week. Massage 1 teaspoon warmed sesame oil into the scalp for 10 minutes before wrapping your hair in a warm towel.

Oily scalp and dry ends can be partially corrected between washings by holding your head upside down and using a wide brush to disperse the natural oil through the hair for 50 strokes.

Coconut Conditioner

All hair and scalp types can benefit from the luxuriant qualities of coconut oil, which is barely scented. Due to the heat in India, women needed to protect their hair from the sun. Coconut oil conditions and nourishes the scalp. Buy a tub (available from Superdrug) and warm in the microwave or in a *bain marie* (a bowl suspended over a saucepan of hot water). Massage your scalp before bedtime and leave the oil on overnight. Use the pads of your fingers to carry out the massage, and smear whatever is left on the rest of your hair. Leave overnight and wash your hair in the morning.

Scalp Friction Massage

Regular scalp massages will help nourish your scalp by increasing oxygen-rich blood flow to the top of your scalp. Hair is more likely to fall out of weary follicles. Massaging makes your scalp less likely to produce dead skin cells, which can lead to dandruff and, in severe cases, psoriasis. There is even evidence that massaging your scalp can help alleviate premature greying and male pattern baldness. It's also extremely pleasant and invigorating, but avoid doing this directly after you have eaten a meal, as the blood is needed for proper digestion. The best time is when you are applying shampoo.

Place the fingers of both hands over the crown of your head and rotate each finger in a small circle. Use a light touch – massaging too firmly will over-activate the sebaceous glands and hair will soon look greasy. Work your way down the back of your scalp. Then place your fingers at the base of your head, just under your skull, before moving around the sides of your head, aiming to cover every inch of your scalp. Make this a way of life, and within a couple of weeks limp hair will start to bounce back. But do brush your hair when it is dry to smooth down any ruffled hair cuticles. (For a more intensive treatment, see the section on Indian head massage, page 94.)

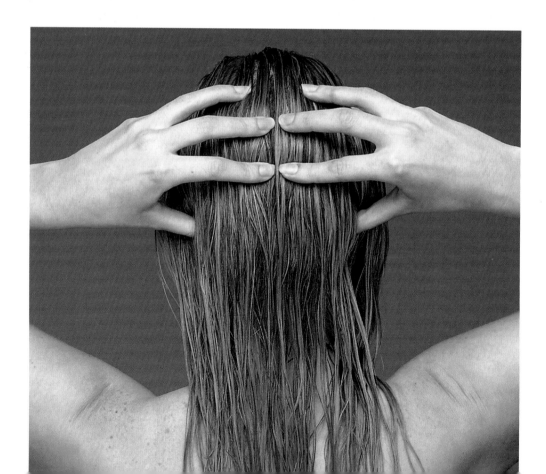

The Secret of Shiny Hair

Each hair is made up of dead protein cells extruded in one direction. The outside of the hair shaft is known as the *cuticle*, and each cuticle is made up of cells like the shiny scales of a fish; smooth to the touch in one direction, but easily ruffled in the other. Hair with a lustrous, shiny glow has a relaxed cuticle, lying flat against the hair shaft. To maintain, don't use very hot or very cold water to wash your hair, don't blow-dry your hair every day, and avoid strong detergent shampoos.

Do brush hair regularly, and use a few drops of lavender oil on the scalp each morning.

Caring for Hair

- Use a gentle, vegetable-based shampoo on your hair and leave it on for up to 10 minutes before rinsing with copious warm water so all dirt will be dissolved.

  Apply conditioner to the ends, not the roots, and comb through with a wide-toothed comb, taking care not to pull or stretch the hair. Don't use too much conditioner, as hair will appear lank; too little and it will remain parched.

- Never brush your hair when it is wet, and don't rub dry with a towel as this will roughen up the cuticle and encourage hair to tangle. Instead, pat dry.

- If hair is tangled, start combing at the ends and gradually work up to the roots, working in small sections at a time and gently coaxing the comb through it.

- If you can, try to avoid using a hairdryer as this encourages hair to dry out. If you do want to use one to style your hair, let your hair dry naturally for at least 20 minutes first.

- Never go to sleep bearing hair clips or ties, as these weaken hair.

- Wear a hat in the sunshine to stop your hair from drying out.

- Avoid using chemical sprays, perming agents or harsh colourants on your hair.

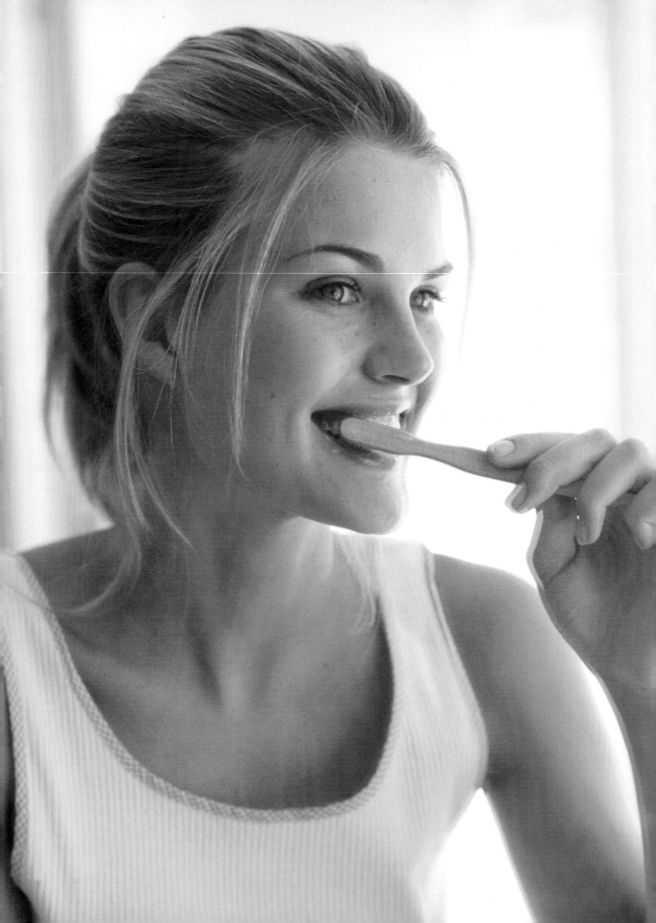

your teeth

I know a highly attractive young man in his thirties who simply refuses to smile in photographs. He fears his teeth will show. Photographs are developed and he looks glum, but if he'd just smile no one would notice his teeth, which are uneven and slightly stained from smoking, and he'd look as happy in pictures as he is in real life. One of my clients, a successful woman in her forties, tends to cup her mouth as she speaks. As she does not have a good sense of smell she fears her breath does not smell good, and she also confided her fears over the fact that her teeth are out of alignment. In fact, her slightly lopsided smile is one of her appealing traits, and there are plenty of ways to overcome bad breath.

Our mouths are full of nerve-endings, so we are subconsciously especially sensitive to what lurks beneath our lips because these are areas rich in sensation. But just because they feel obvious to us doesn't mean our mouths are especially obvious to anyone else. However, loss of confidence in our teeth can be debilitating, even though chances are that the problem is much magnified in your own mind.

The good news is that there is plenty you can do to create a natural attractive smile free from bad breath, discolouration, sensitive teeth and swollen gums. Significantly, make sure you don't smoke and avoid drinking a lot of strong coffee, tea or red wine. Floss and brush effectively. Avoid drinking colas, as these also stain teeth and can swiftly erode and decay them.

While approximately 20 per cent of us have adopted American habits of flossing and using mouthwash, not everyone can afford to follow the US trend for cosmetic dentistry work. However, if you still feel your teeth themselves are the source of your loss of confidence, then refer to Dr Phil Stemmer's dental section in the second part of this book for non-surgical ways to create the perfect smile (see pages 167–173).

teeth and gum health

Sixty years ago, lack of widespread dental care, poverty and a poor diet meant that many people expected to start losing their teeth in their twenties. Today, the number of middle-aged people who need false teeth has dropped from 32 per cent to 6 per cent over the past 25 years, while the days of routine fillings have all but disappeared as fewer children suffer tooth decay. Fizzy drinks, which contain very high percentages of sugar and acid, are our teeth's current biggest adversary, and citrus fruit juices are now considered to be even more damaging than sugar when left on the teeth. If you drink either, try and rinse with water directly afterwards.

Fluoride toothpaste has been a major factor in improving dental health in the UK, as have the minute quantities of fluoride which have been (in some cases controversially) added to tap water in some parts of the UK.

Teeth Tips

Did you know that if you are stressed your teeth can actually decay faster? Stress causes acid to enter your mouth which, like citrus fruit juice, is damaging to your teeth.

Breathe through your nose if you can, as breathing through the mouth causes the protective layer of saliva to dry out, putting teeth and gums under greater risk of attack from bacteria.

Eat foods that are high in vitamins C and D, and calcium – such as dark greens, sea vegetables and high quality dairy produce – to help strengthen the teeth.

Recent research has shown that oolong and green teas can be excellent plaque-reducing aids. They contain *polyphenols*, which inhibit the formation of the bacteria that lead to cavities.

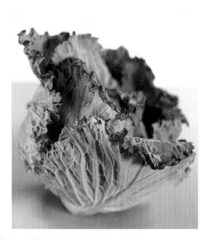

Gargle every day with a few mouthfuls of warm salt water to keep germs and infections at bay (a generous pinch of in half a glass of warm water will suffice).

Chewing a handful of fresh parsley is a tried and tested emergency method of removing the smell of garlic and other strong-smelling foods, but don't rely on this.

Simple Cleaning

Using an electric toothbrush is the kindest thing you can do to your teeth, because it cleans your teeth much more effectively than you could ever do with a toothbrush.

If you do use a normal brush, choose one that is soft and use it in small circles. Never rub side to side, as this can wear down teeth through abrasion. Do remember to clean both inside and outside the rows of teeth, and clean the front teeth as well as the molars at the very back.

Professional cleaning of your teeth, by a dentist or hygienist, involves removing the hard deposits above (supragingival) and below (subgingival) the gum line. These deposits lead to the development of the bacterial colonies that cause gum disease and can lead to decay and loose teeth. Problems with your gums begin below the gum line, so you need to pay attention to this important part of your anatomy.

If your gums bleed when brushed, this is a sign they are infected. Visit your dentist for advice and concentrate on brushing around the gum margins using an angled brush.

Flossing

Flossing is now recommended as the only way to get plaque and food debris out from between your teeth effectively. A lot of people find it difficult or unappealing, but its importance cannot be overstated. Choose waxed floss or tape, which is easier to use. You can also buy floss which is impregnated with tea tree oil, which has a naturally disinfectant quality.

Gum Care

Your gums are often overlooked, but they are vital to your dental health. They help hold teeth in place and they help stop bacteria from destroying the hidden parts of your teeth. Massaging them helps to keep circulation flowing.

Gum Massage Paste

Mix 2 teaspoon rock salt, half a teaspoon black pepper, half a teaspoon turmeric and 1 teaspoon olive oil. Massage the gums in tiny circles to soothe, disinfect and tighten them. Alternatively, massage them with a single fresh strawberry, which helps clean the teeth and has astringent qualities to tone the gums.

your tongue

In traditional Indian and Chinese medicines, the tongue is viewed as an important indicator of health. We completely overlook our tongues in the UK, but try incorporating the following routine into your teeth-cleaning regime to remove the thick grey or white accumulations of unwanted waste and toxins that collect on it: Gently scrape the tongue's surface with the concave tip of a teaspoon, then lightly brush the tongue with the spoon from front to back. Drinking more water helps break down these toxins. A thick layer of residue on the tongue may indicate you are not flushing out your system with sufficient quantities of drinking water. Professionally designed tongue-scrapers are available from Dental Health Boutique (see Resources chapter), and should be used daily.

natural tooth whiteners

Whitening toothpaste can be an effective way of removing staining, but research published in the *British Dental Journal* showed that none of them has the power to change the actual colour of your teeth (they would need to contain an oxidizing agent to achieve that, which they do not). What they can do is remove surface stains, which will superficially improve the appearance of your teeth.

Some are better than others. Dr Phil Stemmer recommends Macleans Whitening toothpaste, which came top in the *British Dental Journal* survey, beating the others by some margin. Aquafresh Whitening came second, and Boots' own whitening brand came third. 'These products contain enzymes and so-called whitening agents which have the power to remove stains with persistent use,' Dr Stemmer explains.

The Boots Advance White Polishing System is a battery-operated tooth polisher that is a good way to remove stains, but you need to use it twice a day for a month before you'll see results. Wrigley's White Orbit gum claims to reduce the build-up of stains by up to 36 per cent when you chew it for 20 minutes after eating.

You can help remove stains from your teeth by cleaning them with half a teaspoon of bicarbonate of soda sprinkled over the damp bristles of your toothbrush. Bicarbonate can remove staining by oxidization, but use infrequently as the bicarbonate contains rough granules which gradually erode dental enamel. 'Using a whitening toothpaste is a safer approach,' cautions Dr Stemmer.

Toothpaste

Use a toothpaste that contains fluoride, and avoid using smoker's toothpaste or toothpaste that feels grainy to the touch. These remove stains, but do so by removing surface enamel, which is only several microns in depth. Eventually you are going to have no enamel, only dentine, which is much, much darker and means you'll be looking at major cosmetic dentistry later in life.

Herbal toothpastes are a fad. 'Companies are bringing out herbal toothpaste just to fill up the shelves and keep rival products off the shelf,' says Dr Stemmer. 'These toothpaste have an organic feel-good factor, but they are of no advantage to your teeth.' He recommends Dentyl pH toothpaste containing soft micro-capsules which burst on brushing, delivering a fresh antibacterial agent beneath the gums.

Toothbrushes

The best investment you can make for your teeth is an electric toothbrush. The British Dental Health Association recommends the Braun 3D, but any oscillating toothbrush is going to be more effective than you twirling a few plastic bristles.

mouthwashes

These can be an excellent way of removing plaque – that amorphous, gelatinous film of bacteria that collects on the teeth and causes tooth decay and gum disease. A tiny amount of bacteria viewed through a microscope is an alarming sight – thousands of tiny wriggling creatures living happily off food debris in the warm conditions of your mouth. It is usually formed when people don't brush and floss teeth regularly. Antibacterial agents are present in mouthwashes and can help eradicate this sticky layer, but avoid using any that contain alcohol. One of the market leaders contains 27 per cent alcohol. Alcohol-based mouthwash has five main drawbacks:

1   It dries the mouth and makes bad breath and gum disease worse.
2   It feeds the bacteria that cause gum disease and bad breath.
3   It dissolves and weakens white fillings.

4   It may increase the risk of oral cancer.

5   It kills or seriously injures approximately 600 children under the age of six every year in the US, when they drink mouthwashes containing alcohol.

Choose a mouthwash that positively declares itself 'alcohol free', as alcohol derivatives go by many different names on ingredient lists.

Bad Breath

Bad breath is evidence that there is an excess of bacteria growing in your mouth, on your tongue, or up under your gums, which give off odorous or unpleasant gases. These gases are often noticeable when you speak or breathe out. Often this is worse after a night's sleep, during which the mouth is often closed, and is called 'morning breath'.

'In over 95 per cent of cases, bad breath comes from the mouth,' says Dr Stemmer, who runs Europe's original Fresh Breath Centre. 'It is very, very rarely from the stomach or from any other medical condition. Bad breath is not, as many assume, an indication that you have a problem with your digestion. Breathe out ... Where is the air coming from, your lungs or your stomach?' Put like that, the answer is obvious. But do bear in mind that other conditions that can contribute to bad breath are illness, low fluid intake, stress, lack of salivary flow and lack of exercise.

Oral malodour mainly occurs from an accumulation of oral bacteria which can live anywhere in the mouth, although usually under the gums, between the teeth, on the palate, between fillings or crowns that don't fit, on the tongue or in the folds of the cheek. If you have a broken filling and food packs underneath, you are likely to get unpleasant breath.

For cases of halitosis (bad breath), your first port of call should be your dentist and hygienist. 'If your gums bleed, that's a sign of disease. It's not normal for gums to bleed. You wouldn't think it normal for your nails to bleed if you washed your hands, and if they did you'd visit your doctor. The same applies to your teeth,' says Dr Stemmer.

Tell-tale signs that you may have bad breath include: Gums that bleed on brushing or flossing, a dry mouth, and/or an unpleasant, metallic taste in your mouth.

It is difficult for anyone to detect whether they have halitosis. The best way is to ask a close friend or family member. Another simple way is to lick your wrist, starting at the back of the tongue and wiping the inner wrist to the tip. Leave the saliva to dry for 10 seconds and smell the area for any unpleasant odours. Most people who think they have a problem will find they do not.

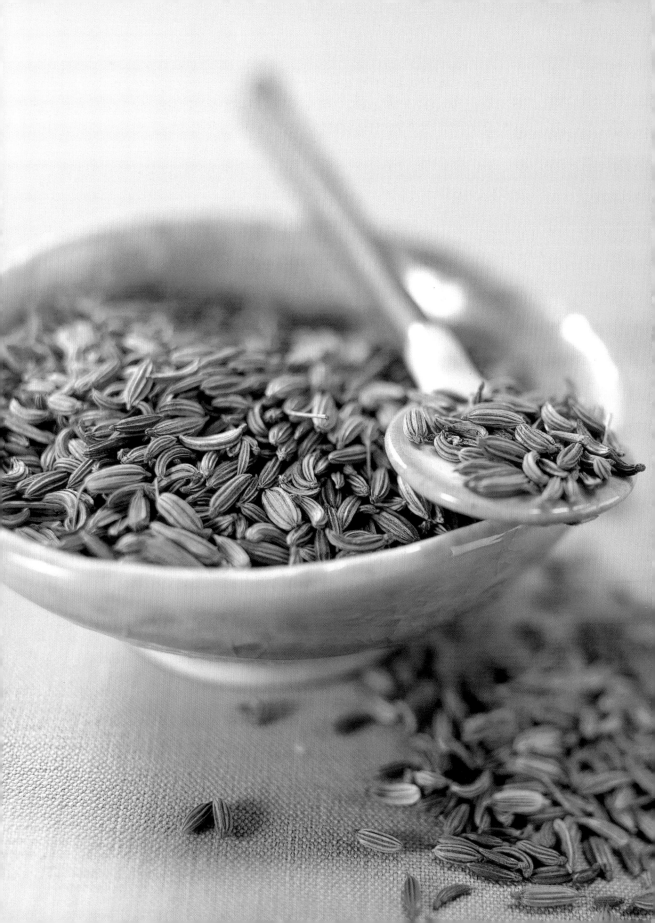

Good oral hygiene is the best way to deal with bad breath:

- Brush properly with an electric toothbrush.
- Use floss correctly – ask your dental hygienist how.

Can Mouthwash Help Cure Bad Breath?

An average of £258 million per year is spent in the UK on mouth-fresheners that do not work or are used incorrectly. They simply disguise one odour with another, stronger odour that lasts no more than 15 minutes. Mouth rinses alone will not solve the problem, but if you do choose to use a mouthwash, one of the most effective is Dentyl pH which came out top of all mouthwashes tested in the US by a non-profit organization, Clinical Research Associates, using volunteer dentists. It actually lifts, absorbs and removes bacteria, dead cells and food debris. You can see it working – when you spit out you can see clumps of debris in the sink. 'Some mouthwashes kill the bacteria, but leave them in the mouth, so the new bacteria eat the old bacteria and they've got plenty of food,' says Dr Stemmer.

Alternatively, chew roasted fennel seeds after meals.

If you are eating strongly-flavoured foods, these can produce temporary bad breath, which can be helped by gargling half a cup of aloe vera juice – but be warned it has a strong bitter taste.

For persistent problems consult the Fresh Breath Centre (details in the Resources chapter).

your eyes

Human beings have evolved as social creatures, and as such our eyes are strategic communication devices. Our coloured iris is set upon a contrasting white background so that we can see precisely, even from a distance, in which direction someone is focusing their attention. Knowing when you talk to someone that their eyes are on you is an important element of creating and maintaining the intricate social connections that define us.

Babies are born with an innate facial recognition centre in the brain – for them, seeing two dots side by side above a line to symbolize the mouth are enough to elicit gurgles and smiles. Rearrange the order of those shapes, put the dots beneath the line for example, and the baby sees only a random pattern without meaning and does not respond. So, from an early age we are programmed subconsciously to focus on each other's eyes. This means that you need only glance in someone's direction to know if they are feeling unwell, over-tired, eating badly, or perhaps drinking and smoking to excess.

The skin around the eyes is mainly serviced by lymphatic vessels which do not have the efficient pumping mechanism of the heart to rely on. Consequently, the delicate tissue around the eye is prone to stagnation, particularly just before a period, when the lymphatic fluid is thicker.

The skin here is the thinnest anywhere on the body, and one of the first places on our face to show signs of ageing because it is not as securely attached to underlying tissue. This means it is sensitive to rough handling. Take special care not to pull or drag the delicate skin around the eyes when washing, cleansing or applying make-up, as this can increase wrinkles.

The underlying tissue is also poorly supplied with sebaceous glands, so using an appropriate, light moisturizer here is important.

Don't overlook the importance to eye health of a good diet, plenty of sleep, exercise, natural light and cutting down on drinking and smoking.

tired eyes

The best way to solve persistently tired eyes is to review your sleeping habits. Check your bed is comfortable, your bedcovers are not too hot or to cold, and that your pillow is giving your neck and head the correct support. Avoid drinking stimulants such as coffee, cocoa, tea or cola after 6 p.m. as they can keep you awake. Exercise for at least 30 minutes every day, but not within six hours of your bedtime. Eat your last meal of the day early so you have time to digest before sleep, and avoid eating cheese or protein-rich snacks before bedtime. Have a warm, scented bath just before you go to sleep to relax body and mind; using 4 drops of lavender oil will help you to unwind. If you worry during the night, keep a pen and paper by your bed and make a list of any sources of stress that are troubling you. If problems of sleeplessness persist for more than two weeks, see a doctor, as this can be an indication of depression.

Eye Massage

One of the best treats you can give your own over-tired eyes is an eye massage, which will help to stimulate the lymphatic system to drain any stagnating fluids or toxins. Apply gentle pressure with the pads of your ring finger around the eye bone, starting in the corner and moving around the elliptical bones that contain the eyes. By doing this you are stimulating a lot of nerve endings, and you will feel a remarkable release of energy. Make 10 laps of the eye, but only use the weaker third finger to maintain a gentle pressure.

See my recipes for eye gel and eye masks (page 47).

Quick Pick-me-up

If you have tired eyes, rest your elbows on a table and rest your face in your hands so that they're covering your eyes. Five minutes will help put the sparkle back.

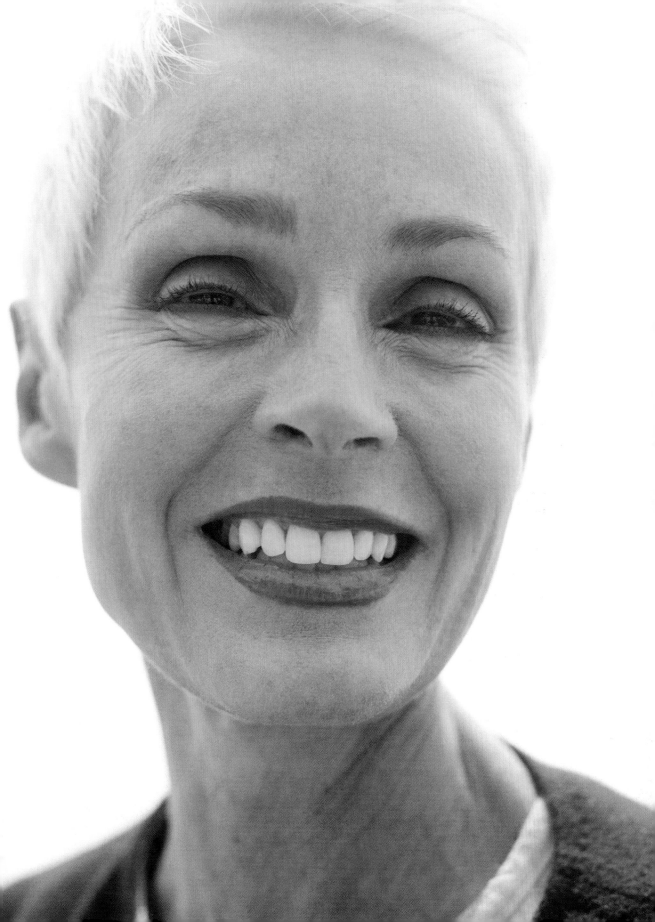

Red Eyes

Avoid using eye-whiteners which are available over the counter. These drops work by narrowing the tiny blood vessels that cover the surface of the eyes, giving the impression of whiter than white whites ... however, when they wear off the blood vessels dilate again and can appear larger than they were before. A vicious cycle beckons. If your eyes are red it is because they are tired, allergic to something, have an infection or are responding to cold or drying winds. Seek medical advice if the problem persists.

Dark Circles or Bags Under the Eyes

If you have dark circles under your eyes, you may have to accept that this is your genetic inheritance due to deep eye sockets, or pale, thin skin revealing the blood capillaries underneath. Dark-skinned people can appear to have dark circles because of excess pigmentation which can be triggered by the deposition of waste products due to a sluggish lymphatic system, causing deeper discolouration.

Blood also tends to pool in the eye sockets overnight, which can intensify the effect. Fatigue, poor diet, lack of exercise and dehydration can all encourage dark circles. Conditions such as eczema and asthma also lead to dark rings. In rare cases, dark circles may indicate the presence of a kidney problem or a nutritional deficiency.

Disguise with a stick concealer, applied under the bags (if you put it on the bags themselves it will highlight them and they will look bigger).

Focus attention on the upper lid by using a richly coloured or dark eye shadow.

If the circles are very dark, disguise using a camouflage foundation with a slightly greenish tone (see page 138).

Eat plenty of foods containing vitamin C and vitamin B_{12}. Boost your diet with leafy green vegetables, beetroot, brown rice, whole grains, beans, blueberries and plums.

Cut down on salt if it makes you retain fluid, and try to identify other foods that may be leading to water retention.

Apply chilled eye gel (see page 47) 15 minutes before making up, and use make-up to draw attention to your upper lids. Use plenty of mascara on the upper row of eyelashes, and give them a curl.

Splash your eyes with cold water on waking.

Sleep on your back to minimize fluid retention under the eyes.

Crow's Feet

Character and experience is etched over time into our faces, and a certain amount of laughter-line wrinkling around the eyes is evidence that you often smile. The key is to keep the delicate skin around the eye from becoming too dry, as not doing so can lead to the lines becoming more deeply etched. Thin skin with little oil becomes dehydrated easily and is more prone to wrinkling.

Drink enough to keep your urine pale yellow.

Use good sun protection.

Eat a good diet.

Use a light, water-based moisturizer every day.

Puffy Eyes

Surprisingly, one of the most common causes of puffy eyes – when the eyelids and surrounding skin swell – is a good night's sleep. When we sleep we don't blink, and this can lead to the build-up of fluid. As we start blinking again – we blink 10,000 times a day on average – the swelling subsides.

Other causes are lack of sleep, sensitivity to skin products, crying, pre-menstrual fluid retention, allergies such as hay fever, and the use of heavy or oily make-up removers which prevent tissue fluids from evaporating naturally overnight. Puffy eyes may also be caused by a thyroid problem, so see your doctor if they persist.

Apply chilled eye gel – or chilled aloe vera gel (see page 47) – 15 minutes before applying make-up. In extreme cases, wrap an ice-cube in a handkerchief and place under the eyes – but for no more than one minute.

Avoid salty foods, and don't add salt to meals.

Choose matt rather than iridescent eye shadow. If your eyes are puffy around the bags, use a slightly darker concealer.

Place a cold, wet flannel over closed eyes for two minutes, followed by a warm one, then a cold one again. This will help boost sluggish circulation.

general eye care

Reading or writing without adequate light, or concentrating on a computer for lengthy periods of time, leads to eye strain which causes vision to blur and eventually deteriorate. Make sure you read only in a brightly-lit place and, if using a computer, give yourself a screen break every 15 minutes where you focus into the far distance for 30 seconds at least. Every couple of hours, give yourself a 10-minute break.

Always wear sunglasses (with UV and infrared protection) in bright sunlight.

An excellent revitalizing tonic for your eyes is milk. Soak a cotton wool ball in milk and apply, when lying down, to your eyelids. Small amounts of milk will seep through onto your eyeball (don't do this if you wear contact lenses, as the milk proteins will upset them). You'll feel refreshed, and these natural eye drops will help the whites of your eyes to look clear.

eyelashes

Eyelashes are one of the most trouble-free areas of your body. Left to their own devices they look after themselves – in fact the only intervention they usually require is a slick of mascara. Eyelash perming is popular in Asia and can really enhance the eyes, but always go to a good salon. It is important that the perming solution is sufficiently weak and applied with due care to this vulnerable area.

If you use eyelash curlers, always use them *before* applying mascara, and consider investing in a pair with soft pads that you can heat with a hairdryer before use, for more dramatic results. Curl twice, once near the root and then halfway down the length of the lash for the most effective results.

Eyelashes can also be salon-tinted with a vegetable colour which will make them appear more glossy and striking, while nourishing the follicle. Avoid using a home-tinting kit, which can be unsafe if not properly applied.

Mascara should be the last item of make-up you apply. Choose an oil-based product that won't end up all over your cheeks. To apply, tilt your head back and stroke onto the underside of the eyelashes. If you want a thicker effect, use a lash-lengthening mascara or put another coat on the top of the lashes. Do not use mascara on the lower lids – the startled spider look is rather old hat – instead, use a smudge of shadow in the outer corner of the lower lashes for a more dramatic effect (see page 139).

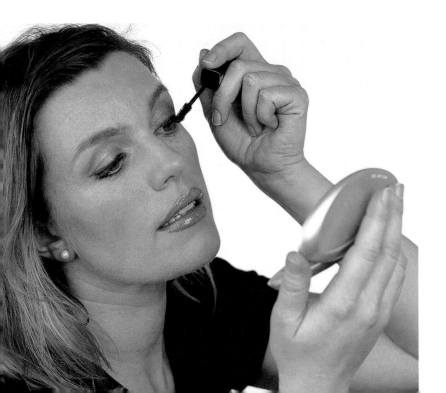

eyebrow shaping

Eyebrows are facial punctuation, making sense of our expressions and lending emphasis to our mood (imagine trying to frown effectively without eyebrows!). Most of the time we overlook our eyebrows, but they can be a great beauty asset, enhancing your best features and limiting the impact of your worst. A well-groomed brow shape itself makes a great unspoken difference to our face – the wrong brows for your facial shape and features can actually spoil an otherwise pretty face.

Leading make-up artist Armand says: 'Eyebrows at the moment are very natural but polished. You want to create a nice even shape that is not too thin, not too wide, but is slightly angular and drawn in a nice arch.' He believes that beautifully defined brows can actually do more for your face than any cosmetic. 'A lot of women ignore their eyebrow shape, which means they are missing a great opportunity to perfect and polish their look. You can have the most stunning eye make-up in the world, but teaming it up with unkempt or un-tweezed brows is like putting a valuable water-colour in a cheap plastic frame. The idea is to give your eyes an almond-shaped look by tidying up the line of the eyebrow.' This will help your face appear slimmer, make your eyes look larger and draw attention away from a heavy chin.

So, time to get 'brow aware'. Unlike other significant changes you may wish to make to your face, you don't need to undergo surgery, inject chemicals or wait months for a change.

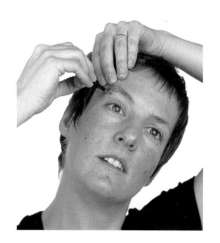

Armed with a pair of tweezers, a steady hand and an idea of what you want to achieve, a whole new look can be yours in minutes. (Also see Make-Up for Brows, page 141.)

Do make sure you choose the right brow shape for your face shape. A highly arched brow is a great way to help a round, jolly face appear longer, but a round brow will make the same face look rounder than ever. The same arched brow on a long face will draw the face out still further.

In Search of the Perfect Brow

Heart-shaped Face

Choose a rounded brow to balance and play down your pointed chin. Avoid a flat brow, which will disrupt the rhythm of your face, making your forehead look heavy and pushing attention down to your chin. (Try 'The Madonna', below.)

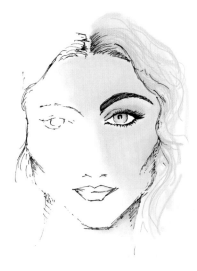

Round Face

Choose an angled brow with a high arch and short tail. Avoid a round brow, which will make you look like a friendly beach-ball. (Try 'The Marilyn Monroe', below.)

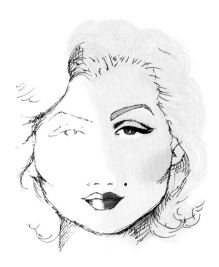

Oval Face

Choose a softly rounded arch to flatter your oval features. Avoid an aggressively arched brow, which will make you look horrified, appalled or perpetually surprised. (Try 'The Grace Kelly', below.)

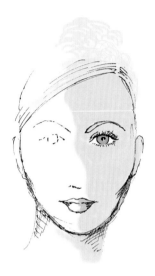

Square Face

Choose a brow that is angled or curved with a sharp peak, which will focus attention away from your jawline. Avoid a delicate, thin rounded shape, which won't have sufficient impact on your strong-featured face. (Try 'The Sophia Loren', below.)

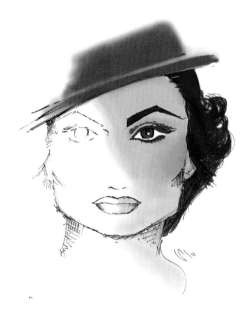

Long Face

Choose a strong, flat brow which will draw attention to your upper face. Avoid an angled brow with a high arch, which will make your face look longer. (Try 'The Audrey Hepburn', below.)

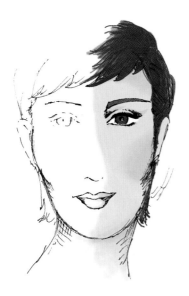

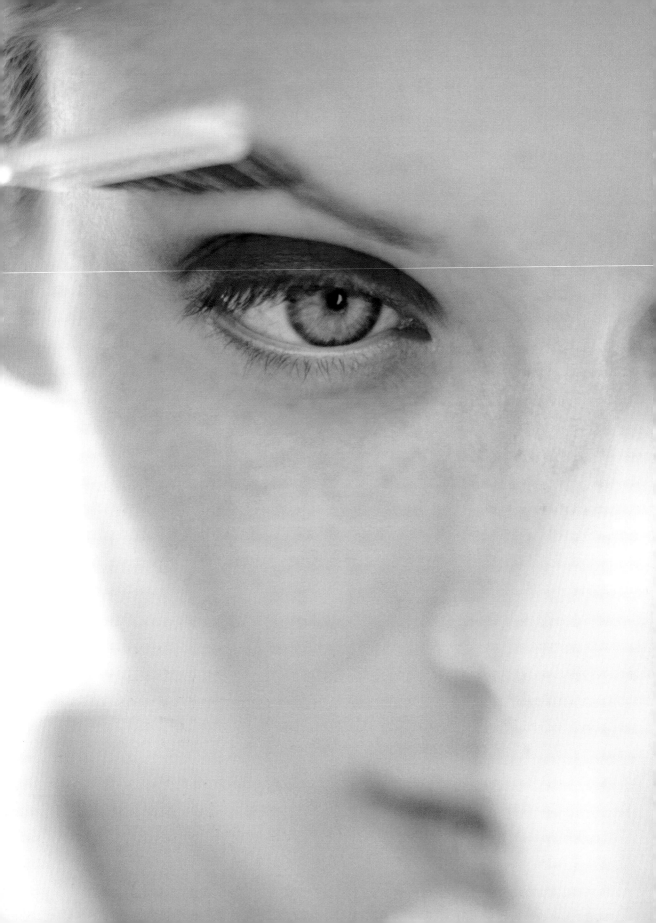

The Five Main Eyebrow Shapes

The Madonna (Round)

Best for an angular or square-jawed face, or for playing down a strong feature on the lower face such as large lips or a strong chin. Like an elegant comma, this is a naturally sophisticated look that is understated yet strong, sculptured yet natural. It draws attention to the upper eye area and gives definition and character.

The Marilyn Monroe (Angled)

Best for a round face. These are super-feminine brows, sensual yet strong, real 'notice-me' voluptuous statements which confer youth and playfulness. The high central peak draws viewers' eyes upwards, but don't overdo it or you'll look artificially surprised. They work well as a foil to other strong features, such as a square jaw. Good for appearing to slim down a wide face.

The Grace Kelly (Soft Angled)

Best for an oval face. These are elegant, understated brows that ooze subtle sophistication. Similar to the Marilyn Monroe, but with a softer, less dramatic arch that looks more gently feminine, not sexually powerful. This is not a statement brow, rather it will work to enhance your other features without drawing attention away from them.

The Sophia Loren (Curved)

Best for a square or oval face or for drawing attention away from a large nose or high forehead. These are bombshell brows that effortlessly ooze sultry sizzle, as well as confidence and professionalism, and are a sensual accompaniment for a strong-featured face. The pointed end of the brow sweeps towards the cheekbones (good for enhancing them if you've got good ones, or for giving your face some structure if you haven't).

The Audrey Hepburn (Flat)

Best for making a long face look more oval, as well as a practical and decisive approach for naturally very heavy brows that would otherwise demand too much attention. These flat brows became Hepburn's signature after she was encouraged to grow them for her title role in *Sabrina*. They are coquettish and playful. Heavy brows like these work on a pixie-like face because they draw attention to the eyes, but they do require careful grooming not to turn into out-of-control caterpillars. Good for enhancing large eyes.

How to Remove Eyebrow Hair

Never use depilatory creams – these can leak into the eyes and cause blindness – also they are not precise enough and you risk dissolving a whole patch of hair.

Shaving

The hair quickly grows back with a blunt end, leaving you with stubble. Only acceptable if your hair is fair or very fine.

Threading

This is a skilled professional approach used in India, and one that I specialize in at my clinic. It involves rolling a piece of cotton thread along the area of unwanted hair. The hairs twist around the thread and, with a deft pull, they are removed by the root, but they must be pulled in the direction of growth. This is *not* something to try at home.

Tweezing

This is a reliable low-tech approach that is the most practical method of all. The best time to pluck is following a hot shower when your skin is supple, the follicle is open and the hair is soft. Make-up artist Armand recommends slicking a touch of Vaseline over the area you plan to pluck to make extraction easier. Alternatively, numb your skin with an ice cube.

Pull in the direction of the hair growth, grabbing the hair just where it emerges from the skin so it does not snap. Tweeze one hair at a time, and be patient. When plucking, you can tweeze hairs from above and below the brow, holding the skin taut while you pluck. It's simply not true that you should never pluck from above – you won't look well-groomed if you have stray hairs there.

Take care when tweezing and don't over-pluck: eyebrow hairs grow back four times more slowly than other body hair, so it can take four to six weeks for a wrongly plucked hair to return.

If you are creating a new shape from a bushy brow, take one hair at a time before turning your attention to its neighbour. Stop, stand back and evaluate every minute or so.

Once brows are shaped, all you need to do is spend a couple of minutes every few days maintaining them. The key is to stay one step ahead of the strays.

The eyebrow follicles are damaged by plucking, which means the hairs are more likely to grow back finer over time. Bear this in mind if you are going for a radical, skinny-brow look you may not wish to retain.

Make-up artist Armand recommends Tweezerman tweezers. 'They are easily the best, but make sure you choose the ones with an angular edge, not a pointed pair, as these make it much easier to get a firm purchase on the hair.'

Laser Treatment

See Nurture section, page 160.

Electrolysis

See Nurture, page 165.

before brow shaping

after brow shaping

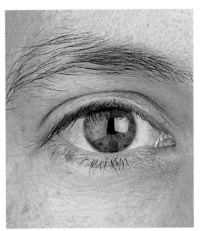
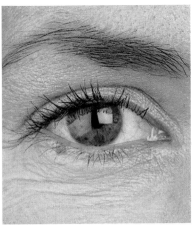

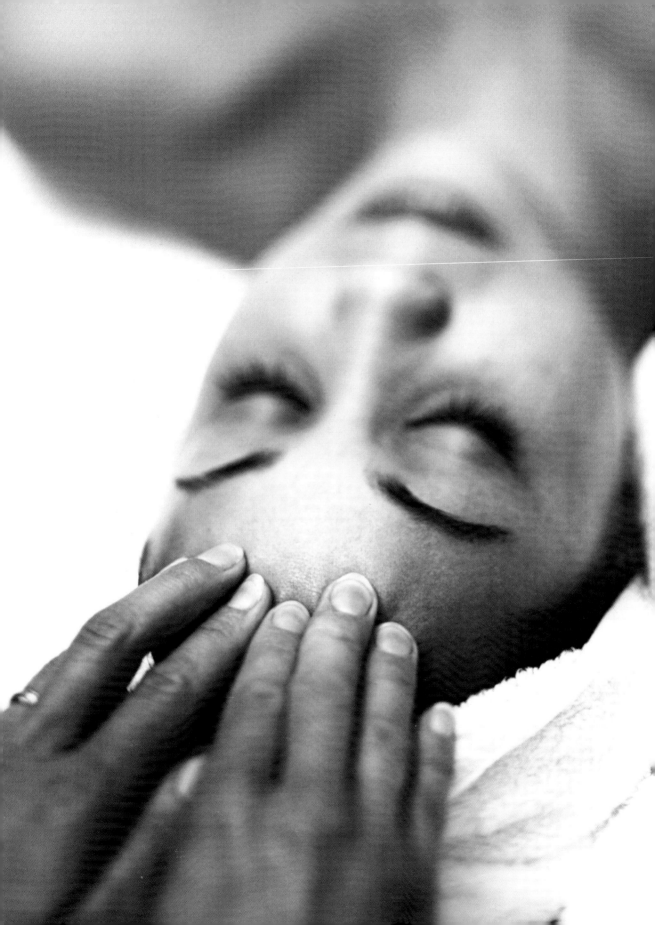

facial massages and exercises

The face and scalp are crowded with nerve endings, which makes them extremely receptive to touch, but usually they are overlooked beyond a brisk rubbing in of shampoo a few times a week. As babies we are frequently touched on our faces – touch is essential for stimulating our nervous system and promoting healthy physical development, but as we grow older, and in the absence of an attentive lover, the temptation is to forget this.

Yet when you go to the hairdresser and receive even the most cursory of 'head massages', you can immediately feel the deeply sensual and soothing benefits of this deep, tension-freeing experience.

Our faces are constructed of a complex arrangement of approximately 120 muscles which help us chew, blink and express ourselves. Yet how often do most people ever think of exercising them? The tendency is to expect them to work perfectly in the absence of any support.

In this chapter I am going to tell you all you need to know to pamper, stimulate, invigorate and exercise your face and head through exercises, massage and acupressure. One of the most wonderful things about massage is that, being formalized, it gives you permission to touch and be touched within established boundaries. You can use these techniques on anyone you know. However, I am presenting them as self-care techniques which you can choose to adapt – if you wish to share their secrets!

bharti's clearing head and scalp massage

This is one of the most delightful therapies you can give yourself. It is a safe, simple and effective therapy that promotes hair growth, as well as providing relief from stress.

Your scalp has an enormous number of nerve endings, blood vessels and acupressure points. In Ayurvedic terms the head chakra – the point right at the top of the head – is known as the white chakra and is called 'the seat of peace'. Other important chakras are located in the brow and the neck. While Western science doesn't recognize chakras, it is known that certain hormone-producing glands lie at the same levels. Whatever language you use, head massage aids well-being.

This is also an effective way to deal with headaches. Tension headaches are caused when the hormone adrenaline floods our system and constricts the blood vessels. Migraine is caused by tension in the eyes, leading to a similar constriction of blood vessels. Massage can effectively re-stimulate the blood vessels so that they relax and help the circulation to normalize.

Head massage has been an important part of Indian family life for more than a thousand years. It began as a grooming technique, when women would use it to spread oil through the hair in order to keep it strong and lustrous. Meanwhile, barbers used to massage their male clients, cutting hair and then offering 'champi' or head massage to invigorate and stimulate the scalp. The derivation of the word 'shampoo' is 'champi'.

Today, Indian babies often receive a daily massage from birth. From three to six years old they are massaged once or twice a week. After the age of six they share massage with other family members on an equal footing. My six-year-old granddaughter Serena loves to give massages. When her mother Priti suffers with a headache, Serena always volunteers to give her a clearing head and scalp massage.

If you are feeling stressed, angry or overworked, tension accumulates in the neck, shoulders and head. The temptation is to take a painkiller to block the pain 'messages', but this is merely a cover-up and will not change the situation. Indian head and scalp massage uses a firm rhythm to release this tension on both a physical and spiritual level by tackling the problem at its source – relaxing the tense muscles that cause the problem.

I grew up with head massage and I later came to realize that the therapy could bring relief from aches and pains all over the body, as scalp massage stimulates acupressure points that affect the entire body.

Massage helps to drain away toxins that accumulate in your skin and muscles, and it improves your circulation. It can also provide help for disturbed sleep and insomnia. Regular massage improves the tone and texture of the skin. Massaging the head also helps to spread the skin's natural oils along the entire hair shaft, which means you won't have to rely so much on conditioning treatments. But most importantly, scalp massage helps to nourish the hair follicles by improving circulation and encouraging waste to drain away, which improves the quality of the hair.

The Two Basic Massage Techniques
Rubbing

Using fairly firm pressure, the balls of your fingers lock onto the skin and move it loosely over the bones of the scalp.

Friction

Your hands glide firmly over the surface of the skin or hair, as if you were trying to rub away a mark.

Using Oil

I always use coconut oil, which leaves hair wonderfully glossy. It is solid at room temperature, so you will need to liquefy it before use in a *bain-marie*. It is also much better applied warm. Coconut oil can be difficult to find so try chemists or healthfood shops; a good alternative is sesame oil. If your skin is particularly sensitive, use olive oil.

Depending on the condition of your scalp you may wish to add a few drops of the following oils:

For greasy hair	Camomile, lemongrass
For dry hair	Ylang ylang, sandalwood
For itchy scalp	Cedar wood, tea tree
For dandruff	Patchouli, tea tree

The Technique

Because our scalp is covered by our hair, we don't see its real condition. If you have a scalp condition, give yourself a massage every day. For basic maintenance, once a week is sufficient. Your goal is the creation of lustrous, shiny, healthy hair through nourishment of the follicle.

Using the friction technique to stimulate the scalp and get that circulation flowing will confer the same benefits as hair products, but via a completely different approach: removing any stagnation in the underlying dermal layer which is affected by hormones, and encouraging nutrients into the scalp with increased blood flow. But head massage alone isn't enough, you need to ensure you are drinking plenty of water and eating a nutrient-rich diet.

Let me show you the technique taught to me by my mother, and which I have taught my daughters and granddaughters.

1   Place your fingertips on your hair line and make tiny, firm, rubbing circles so that the skin moves over the underlying bone (I call these 'fingerballs'). Continue to move around the hair line, following round past the ear on the protruding bone and on into the nape of the neck where the majority of nerves enter the spine.

2   Take hold of your hair in a series of handfuls if it is short, or gather it into a high ponytail if long. Give it several firm tugs to awaken the scalp in preparation for oiling.

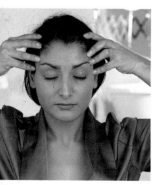
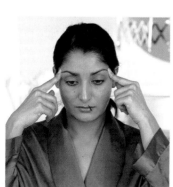
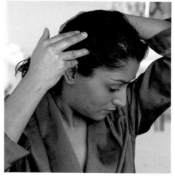
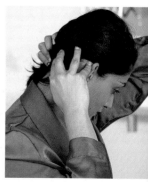

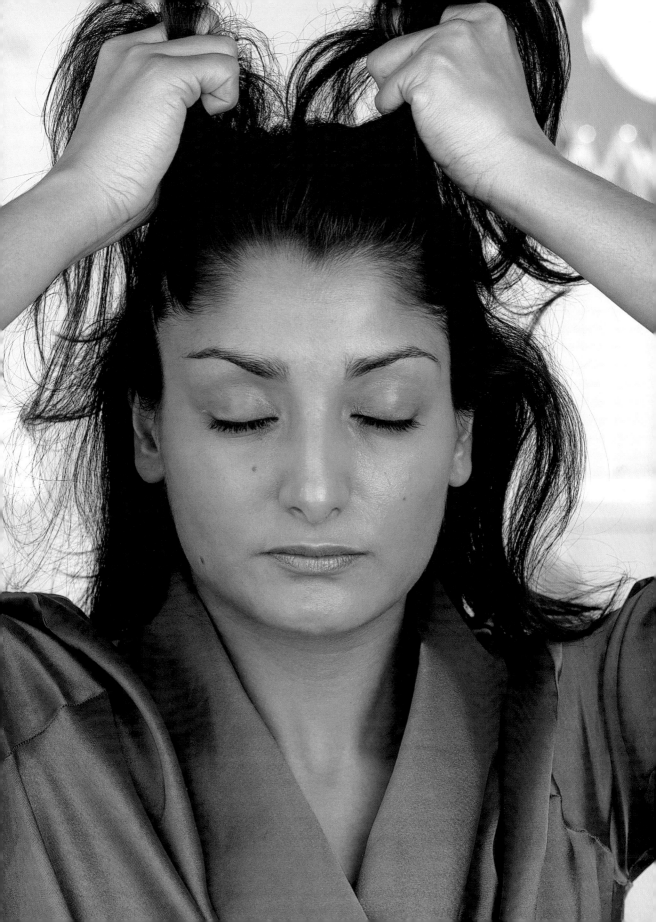

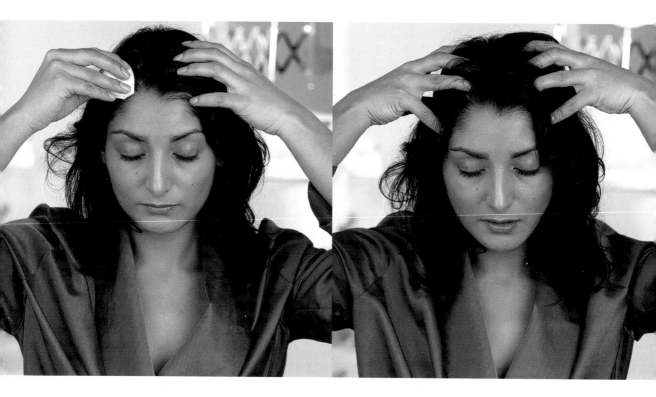

3   Pour your chosen oil (see above) into a shallow bowl. Take a cotton wool ball and soak it in the oil, lightly squeezing out any excess so it doesn't drip. Part your hair in the middle and mop the cotton wool into the parting, and use your fingertips to rub the oil lightly into the scalp. Repeat this all over the head so the entire scalp is oiled.

4   The top of the head is the most important area as it has five powerful acupressure points. These help balance emotions, raise energy levels, sharpen mental faculties and improve memory and concentration. Use your palm in a vigorous sideways flicking action, gliding over the surface of the scalp. Alternatively use your fingertips in a vigorous backwards and forwards friction motion as if applying shampoo rapidly. This doesn't have to be particularly deep, but make sure you cover the entire scalp, nape and neck. Do this for at least 2 minutes.

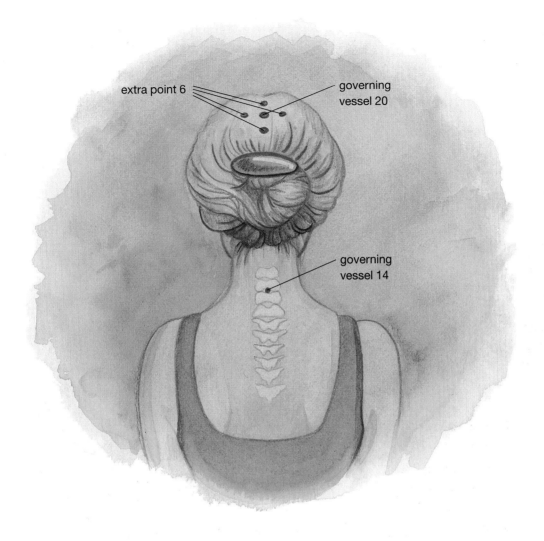

extra point 6

governing
vessel 20

governing
vessel 14

5   Dig in and use rubbing but soothing fingerballs to massage, firmly and persuasively, each part of the scalp. This is a pressure massage, similar to the massage you gave your hairline at the beginning of the treatment. Do this for at least 2 minutes.

6   Once again, pull the hair to awaken the scalp.

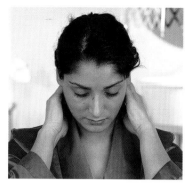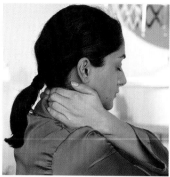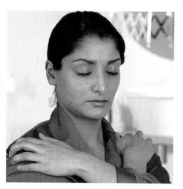

7   Wrap your arms across your chest and over the muscles between your shoulder and neck. Dig in with your fingertips, both sides of the neck muscles. Pinch firmly. Then move along and over the shoulders and down the upper arms, focusing on the deltoid muscles, and repeat. Don't overlook this stage. The head rests on the neck, which is in turn supported by the shoulders. Slouching upsets the balance, but this treatment can help.

Ideally, the entire massage should take 15 minutes and will help relax you, relieve anxiety and help clear your thinking. For the best benefits for your hair leave the oil on for at least a further 15 minutes while you have a bath, but overnight if possible.

Sharing the Massage

This massage is a wonderful gift to give your partner, but do encourage them to return the favour so you will have the energy and inclination to continue treating each other.

Choose a warm, draught-free location with soft lighting or candlelight. Your subject should sit in a straight-backed chair with their legs uncrossed, feet flat on the floor and hands resting in their lap. Ask them to remove any jewellery or hair ornaments. Stand behind them. Take a few deep breaths to relax yourself. Invite them to close their eyes.

acupressure treats

Acupressure is a self-care technique for promoting health. The application of fingertip or thumb pressure at specific points on the body is a popular Chinese approach to health care, and I have found it a very valuable beauty tool. Here are three of the most powerful points on the head which can provide a real pick-me-up whenever you are feeling weary. Treat each acupressure point by applying, then releasing, a deep pressure. Carry out this 'pumping action' once a second for one minute, to activate its curative potential.

For Emotional Balance

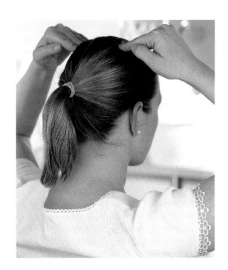

Name	Extra Point 6
Where	Two finger-widths from the middle of the top of the head, to the right and left
How	Apply pressure with the index and middle fingers of each hand
Benefits	Balances the mind, relieves anxiety and insomnia

For a Crick-free Neck

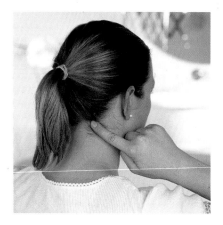

Name	Gall Bladder 20
Where	At the back of the neck, just above the hairline in the depression between the bottom of the skull and the neck muscles
How	Apply pressure with both your index fingers
Benefits	Relieves stiffness and discomfort in the neck and shoulders

For Clearer Thinking

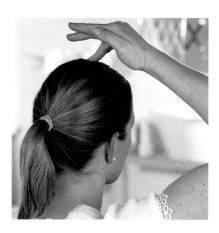

Name	Governing Vessel 20
Where	In the middle of the top of the head, halfway between the ears
How	Apply pressure using index finger
Benefits	The most powerful sedative point in the body. Balances emotions and sharpens mental faculties, as well as improving memory and concentration. Very effective at regulating blood pressure and raising general energy levels.

facial lymphatic massage

Lymph is barely understood, but it holds the key to firmer, smoother skin and enhanced health. When lymph flows easily the skin appears firm and smooth. Any congestion, leading to an accumulation of waste, renders our skin swollen and puffy. When the system is working properly, 2 litres of lymph is cleansed and purified every day.

The lymphatic system has its work cut out for it just conducting daily maintenance. When we are ill, its workload increases. If your lymph nodes (glands) feel swollen, that's a sign the system is working overtime. Drinking too much alcohol or coffee, eating starchy foods overloaded with additives, smoking or over-exposure to pesticides all overload the system, eventually leading to cellulite in certain areas.

What Is Lymph?

The lymphatic system is the body's primary disease-fighting mechanism, but most people are barely aware of its existence. Alongside our arteries, veins and capillaries there is a separate, but connected, network of lymphatic channels. The skin, fatty tissue and muscles are bathed in a sea of lymph. It is similar to blood in every way, but contains no red blood cells. Unlike the blood-containing vessels, these ducts open directly into the tissue spaces between the cells because, as well as fighting infection and repairing damage in every area of the body, the lymphatic network is also our body's vital combined sewage and drainage system, working constantly to remove debris, foreign bodies and excess fluids from the spaces between the cells. When the lymphatic system breaks down it can cause many distressing conditions such as asthma, eczema, sinus trouble, cystitis, bronchitis, laryngitis, arthritis, ear and eye problems.

In his book *Get Well, Stay Well*, Dr Paul Sherwood writes:

Lymph is the name given to the fluid that passes along the lymphatic vessels towards the nearest group of lymph nodes, so that any dead cells, foreign or toxic substances can be filtered out and destroyed by the white blood cells before the fluid is returned to the veins. Each set of lymph nodes (commonly called glands) is responsible for draining a particular area of the body, and are strategically placed around the body to act as centres for the production of antibodies against invading bacteria or viruses carried to them from the tissue spaces.

This explains why swollen lymph nodes in a particular area are such a useful tool for diagnosing infection.

Lymphatic drainage for the face is like a powerful little holistic face-lift. Using a featherlight touch along the lymphatic channels can help to clear areas of congestion and stagnation. A clinic-based treatment is the most effective approach, as your therapist understands fully the lymphatic structure, but a basic facial massage is a helpful home treatment.

'Simple massage techniques are extremely effective in assisting lymphatic flow and drainage,' says Dr Sherwood.

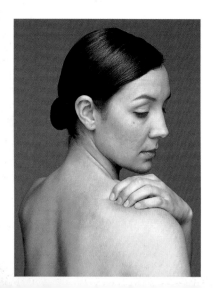

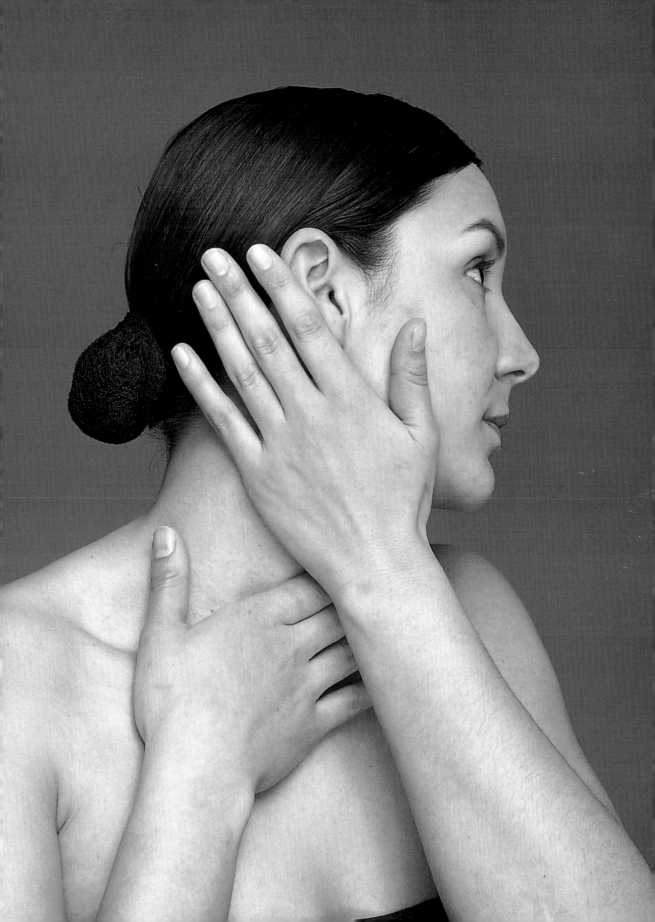

how to give yourself a facial massage

My holistic approach to treatment typically doesn't deal with specific areas in isolation, and so I always include the neck, ears, chest and hands in my weekly facial lymphatic massage. During the massage you will be using the palms (calming and draining), flats of four fingers together (to disperse fat) or your fingertips (concentrated drainage and fat dispersal).

This massage should take between 10 and 15 minutes – any longer and you risk over-stimulation.

1   Before beginning the massage it is important to polish the skin to remove dead cells.
2   Oil the face, neck and chest with almond oil.
3   Begin working on your chest. Cross your arms over your chest and use the flats of your palms with a firm pressure of strokes, moving slowly up across the chest towards the neck, a little at a time. Each stroke should begin with a firmer pressure, decreasing through the stroke until it is almost a feather touch. Aim for continuity in rhythm and intensity, and balance the number of strokes applied to each side of the body. If you are feeling tense in any area, linger there a while.

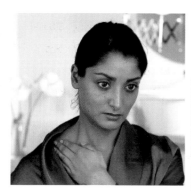
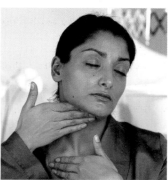
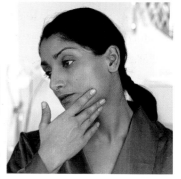

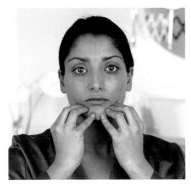
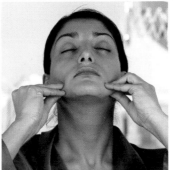
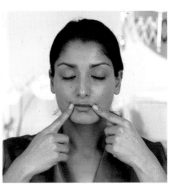

4   You will by now have worked up to the jawline. Push the palms up towards the ears on the underside of the jawline, and bring them over the top of the jaw and back down towards the chin to help break up fat deposits.

5   Place all fingers firmly on the chin. Pinch and hold with the thumb underneath the chin.

6   Move the pinch up around the jawline, squeezing firmly as you go, without dragging the skin. This will help to help disperse fatty tissue, encourage lymphatic circulation and ease any accumulated tension being carried in the jaw. Go as far as the joint of the jaw, then return back down to the neck.

7   Place the thumbs firmly underneath the tip of your chin and rest your index fingers just above your top lip. Firmly brush your fingers in a heart shape around your mouth.

8   Place your tongue under your lip line to make it taut. Lightly pull your index finger around your lip line to tighten the skin slightly while massaging in tiny circles over the lip line with your middle finger. This will invigorate the circulation, bring colour to your lips, discourage the formation of wrinkles and encourage the elimination of oil and blackheads next time you wash. Pay extra attention to the often neglected corners of your mouth.

9   There is a tendency to develop blackheads on the oilier central panel of the face. This technique will help to loosen any plugs of oil blocking pores on and around your nose. Place your index finger in the dimple at the side of the base of your nose. Make tiny circles up the side of your nose, eventually sweeping up over the bridge and pulling your finger down firmly onto the tip of your nose.

10   Move up the nose and onto the sinus areas, making small circles with your index fingers, then up between the eyebrows and on to the forehead.

11   Move out across the forehead using a combination of single-finger and four-finger strokes.

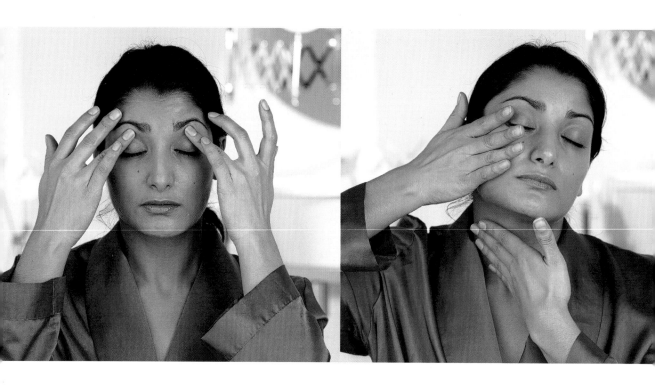

12 On the temples, press and release several times, then make a slow and sustained circular movement using quite deep pressure.

13 Take your palms back onto your cheeks and make sweeping motions back towards your ears.

14 Place your palms on your forehead, starting in the middle and moving them both on one side towards your temples, overlapping your strokes. Travel back to the centre and repeat for the other side.

15 Place your ring finger on the inner edge of your eye socket and make tiny pressured movements as you slowly travel around the sockets in the direction of your ears, to encourage lymphatic flow.

16 Take off earrings if you are wearing them. Pinch your lobe between your thumb and index finger and rub your ear between your fingers, travelling up the hard ridge of the outer ear.

17 Fold the ear over the ear hole, and use your thumbs to massage the cartilage of the back of the ear firmly, moving up and down several times. Repeat on the inner ear.

18 Finally, massage your hands, which will have a coating of oil from your face. Pinch with the thumb and index finger of the other hand deep down into the pockets between the fingers. Pull sharply on each finger. Massage intensively along the length of each finger. Finish by massaging your wrists, using firm strokes from your thumb.

Facial Acupressure Treats

There are certain powerful acupressure points on the face that assist the whole body. Here are some of my favourite and most invigorating ones.

For Releasing Sinus Blockages

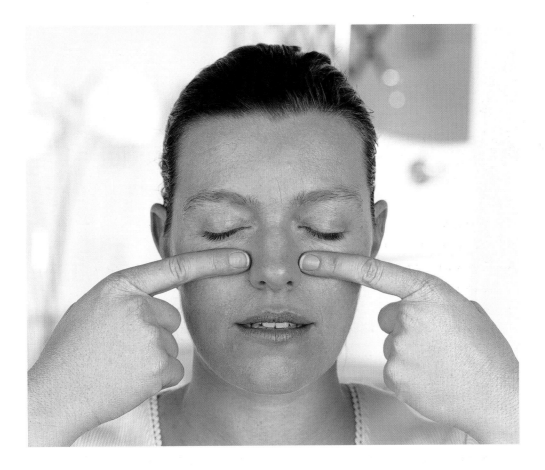

Name	Large Intestine 20
Where	At the groove on the outside edge at the bottom of the nose
How	Press gently against the bone of the nose with the middle or index fingers
Benefits	Massaging the area around the nose helps release sinus blockages and improves the complexion

Wakey Wakey

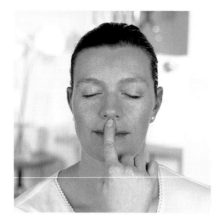

Name	Governor Vessel 26
Where	Just above the middle of the upper lip, above the pout
How	Apply continuous firm pressure with the fingertip of the index or middle finger (stop if you feel unwell, and avoid if you have high blood pressure)
Benefits	Tones the facial muscles, improves mental alertness and stimulates the gums

Facial Toner

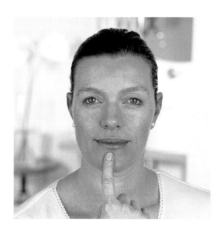

Name	Conception Vessel 24
Where	Just below the middle of the lower lip
How	Apply continuous firm pressure, pressing slightly upwards, towards the lower lip with the index or middle finger
Benefits	Tones the facial muscles and skin and improves the saliva flow

Winter Warmer

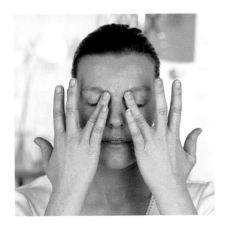

Name	Urinary Bladder 2
Where	Just under the eyebrow on the inner edge of the eye socket
How	Apply pressure with the thumbs pressing upwards against the bony socket of the eye
Benefits	Brightens the eyes and clears the nasal passages

A Tonic for Alertness

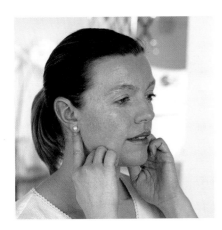

Name	Gall Bladder 2
Where	Just behind the jaw bone and in front of the ear lobe in the depression formed when the mouth is open
How	Rest the thumbs against the jawbone and locate the point with the middle or index fingers, then apply pressure behind the top of the jaw bone
Benefits	Improves hearing and helps maintain healthy teeth and gums

Massaging the chakra known as 'the third eye' – a bundle of nerves in the centre of the forehead, also known in acupressure as Governor Vessel 23 – gives the face an invigorating energy boost.

Stroking the cheeks close to the ears helps to coax stagnant lymph down towards the nodes in the neck.

Signs of Lymph Congestion

Cellulite

Under-eye puffiness

Persistent sinusitis

Pasty complexion

Frequent colds

Inability to fight off infection

Recurrent catarrh

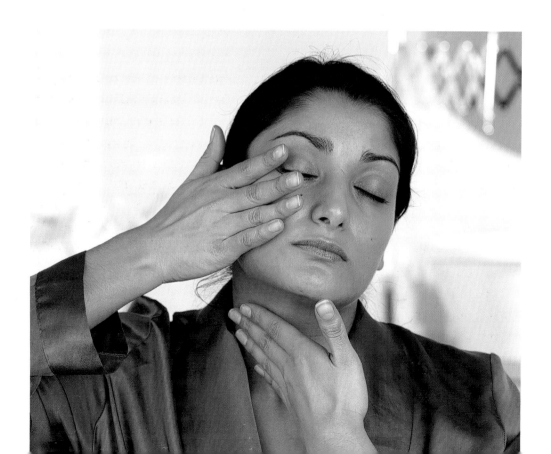

facial exercises

Take a moment to look honestly at your facial 'greeting' – the natural expression of your face in repose that you present to the world. Often when we look in a mirror to check our appearance we smile, or assume an expression that flatters our faces. But in daily life, away from that mirror, we forget about this self-flattering behaviour and relax our facial muscles into the expression that we wear 80 per cent of the time. Look into a mirror with your eyes closed and assume the expression you wear when driving a car or reading a book. Now, open your eyes. Is this you? Or rather, is this the you that you feel you want to project? All too often our relaxed expression is a limited, closed-in version of ourselves that does nothing to express our inner *joie de vivre*.

You cannot alter your underlying bone structure, but you can affect the tone of your facial muscles. Our faces contain 120 different muscles. Their condition is a major determinant of how we look. Their bulk, shape and tone contribute to the structure and contours of our face. As certain emotions register, the patterns of use of our muscles are habituated. By adulthood our patterns of expression tend to be fixed. Some muscles are over-used and others desperately underused. This leads to a decline in definition, both in our expressive abilities and in the apparent youth of our faces. Some facial muscles are attached to bone, others to the skin itself. Often what we call 'natural ageing' is partly due to poor muscle tone in the underpinning of the skin – a regularly exercised face retains its definition and sculptural contours, however old we are.

Exercising your face by working out the underlying muscle helps you to look relaxed, fit, glowing and youthful, and can make significant changes to your expression in repose. Repeatedly contracting and relaxing any muscle – including those in the face – boosts circulation and improves the condition of the overlying skin. It helps disperse a surplus of fat, reduces fluid retention in the exercised area, prevents unnecessary tension and makes you feel brighter and better by raising your endorphin levels (the body's natural feel-good chemicals which are stimulated by any form of exercise). And, as in other forms of exercise, stretching the facial muscles is also important. Face stretches release tension and can help reduce stress.

Simple Stretching Exercises

Stretching Exercise 1: Relaxing a Vertical Frown

Place the tip of your thumb on the inside corner of one eyebrow. Place your index finger on the inside edge of the opposing eyebrow. Keeping good contact with the skin, gently pull the skin sideways until you feel resistance. Completely relax the underlying muscle, and make a mental note of how the exercise feels. Hold for 10 seconds. When you are stressed or worried, make a conscious effort to remember how this sensation felt, and then try and mimic this by using your muscles alone.

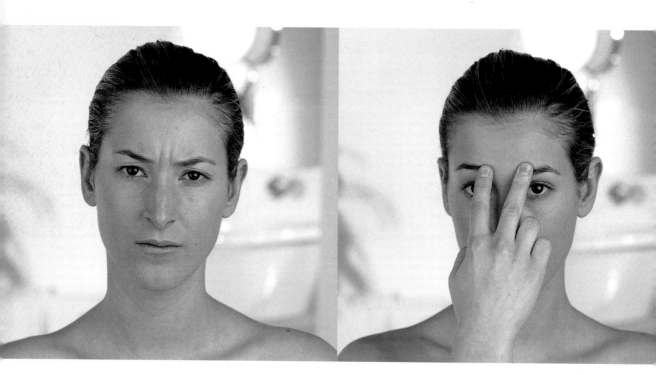

Stretching Exercise 2: Relaxing a Horizontal Frown

Place the tip of your middle fingers on the bottom edge of your forehead above the inside corner of your eyebrows. Place your index fingers above your middle fingers at the top of your forehead, just below the hairline. Keeping good contact with the skin, gently pull the skin vertically until you feel resistance. Completely relax the underlying muscle, and again, make a note of how the exercise feels. Hold for 10 seconds. When stressed or worried, and likely to frown, remember how this sensation felt and try to mimic it using your muscles alone.

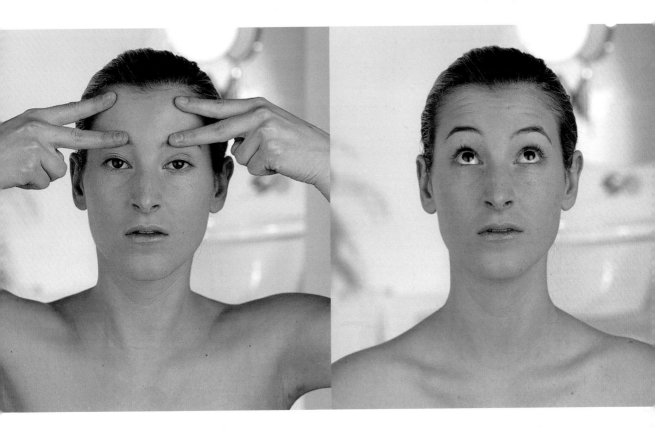

Stretching Exercise 3: De-stressing Your Mouth

The last time you'll have tried this oral tension-relieving exercise was probably at primary school. But it's a very effective way to counteract tension. Open your mouth as wide as you can and make a variety of loose 'rubber mouth' expression for 20 seconds.

Stretching Exercise 4: Giving Your Neck a Workout

Help to prevent a double-chin or tighten up a sagging neck by exercising the long strap muscles either side of your wind pipe. Sit with your shoulders back and square. Turn your head as far as it will go to the left, and then to the right, holding in each position for 3 seconds. Return to the centre and raise your chin up as far as is comfortable; hold for 3 seconds. Then turn your head gently and slowly from side to side as far as is comfortable, holding for 3 seconds either side. Repeat three times. This exercise will also help keep your neck supple.

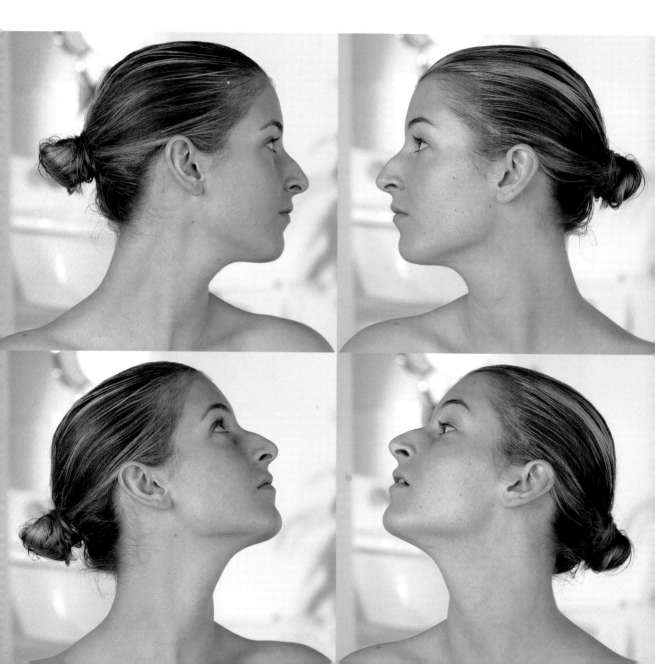

Facial Toning

Tips

As you complete the next few exercises, remember to breathe deeply. Don't hold your breath.

If you are exercising an area that has fine lines you are concerned about over-animating, plant a fingertip gently on the area to keep the skin still while you exercise the underlying muscle only.

If your skin feels taut or tight, apply moisturizer before exercising.

Use gentle movements. Your facial muscles are small, and will feel the benefit even of gradual toning.

Be aware that facial exercises to remove tension may make you feel uneasy. You are letting go of stress which may have been deeply held, and this may lead to old memories, pangs and stiffness emerging. Persist, so that your face is re-animated from underneath its habitual mask.

Relax your jaw. Many of us hold our jaw forwards to keep our mouth closed. Allow it to relax completely when doing these exercises. Your mouth may open slightly. Allow the tip of your tongue to rest on the upper palate behind your front teeth.

For a more intense effect, stimulate acupressure points before you exercise to help drain away accumulated stress (see pages 101–2).

When completing the facial exercises it can be difficult to understand exactly which of the 120 facial muscles is being targeted. With each exercise I've suggested a facial expression you should pull and relax, before starting, so you can feel the muscle concerned in isolation.

Toning Exercise 1: Anti-squinter

Vertical lines between the eyebrows are a common response to habitual stress and pensiveness.

To locate the *corrugator supercilii* muscle, look dissatisfied (see below). You will feel your eyebrows being pulled together by the muscle. You want to encourage this muscle to relax.

- Place two fingers on the inside corner of your eyebrows either side of your nose.

- With your eyes open, use the muscle between your eyebrow to draw your fingers together.

- Now use your eyebrow muscles to send your fingertips as far apart as you can, by lifting up and out.

- Repeat 10 times without your fingers in position.

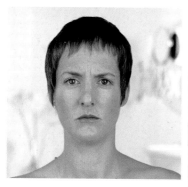
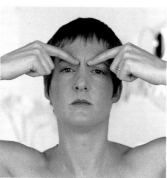
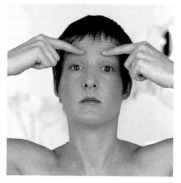

Toning Exercise 2. Toning Your Upper Eyelid

A lazy, untoned upper lid is a common response to a lack of expressiveness.

To locate the *orbicularis oculi* muscle, look surprised (see below). You will feel your eyebrows lift high, pulling on the eye area. You want to encourage this muscle to work harder.

- Gently place your fingertips just above your eyebrows and press down gently. Close your eyes.

- Stretch upwards with your eyebrows as far as you can, while simultaneously pushing your eyelashes as far as you can towards your mouth, using the muscles of your eyelid to pull the skin of your upper lid taut over your eyeball.

- Hold for a count of 5, then slowly relax.

- Repeat 8 times without your fingers in position.

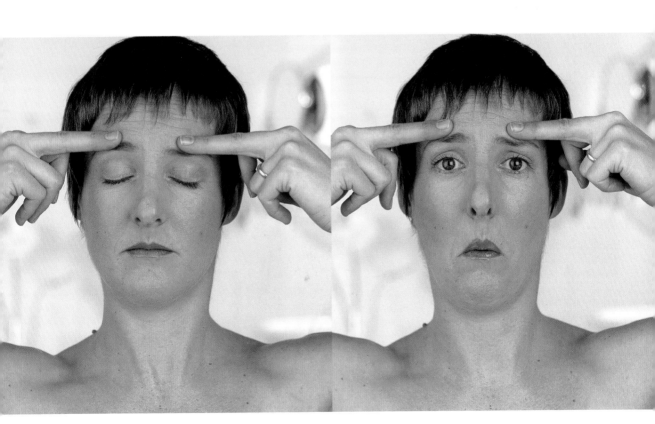

Toning Exercise 3: Smoothing Deep Smile Lines

Lazy muscles can develop around the mouth, leading to deep lines between the nose and chin either side of the mouth.

To locate your *levator quadratus labii superioris* muscles, look disgusted as if you have just smelled something unpleasant (see below). You will feel your nose wrinkle, pulled up by muscles just at the top of the smile line.

● Gently place your fingertips above your eyebrows.

● Flare your nostrils as wide as possible and raise your eyebrows high and wide against the resistance of your fingers. Wrinkle up your nose as much as you can, imagining it moving upwards towards your forehead.

● Use the muscles in your upper lip to pull your nose down towards your chin while keeping up the resistance of your raised eyebrows.
Repeat 10 times without using your fingers.

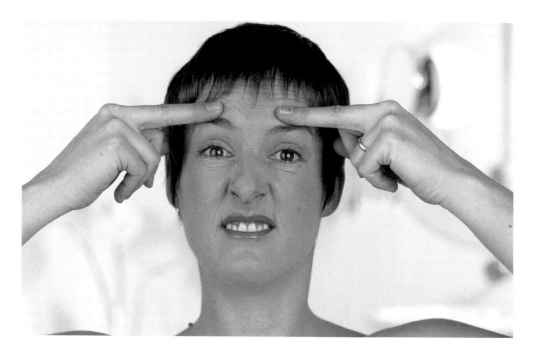

Toning Exercise 4: Toning the Lower Cheeks

One effect of ageing is that we often develop saggy jowls as the muscles relax and lose their elasticity, barely working at all.

To locate your *zygomaticus major* and *minor* muscles, fill your mouth with air as if you are a child about to explode the air out through your mouth (see below). This is now exactly what you're going to do, cheek by cheek.

- Fill up one cheek with air and force the air through your closed lips. The air provides 'resistance-training' for your cheek if you only let a tiny amount seep out.
  Repeat until the cheek muscle feels tired, then swap over to the other cheek.

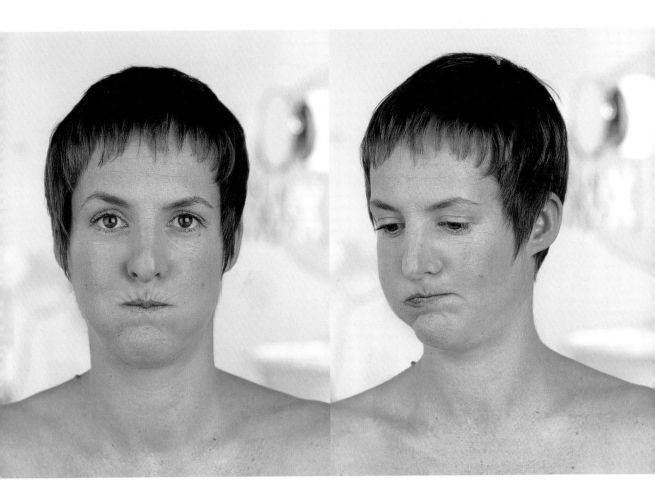

Toning Exercise 5: Sharing Joy

As we age we can forget to smile, and in time our mouths and lower cheeks droop. This exercise will help create a happy cast to the corners of your mouth.

To locate your *zygomaticus major* and *minor* muscles, smile as widely as you can. They are located just under the apple of your cheeks (see below).

- Smile widely, then force yourself to widen the smile still further, raising your eyebrows high and wide, lifting up the corners of your mouth and stretching out your upper lip.

- Gently relax.

- Repeat 10 times.

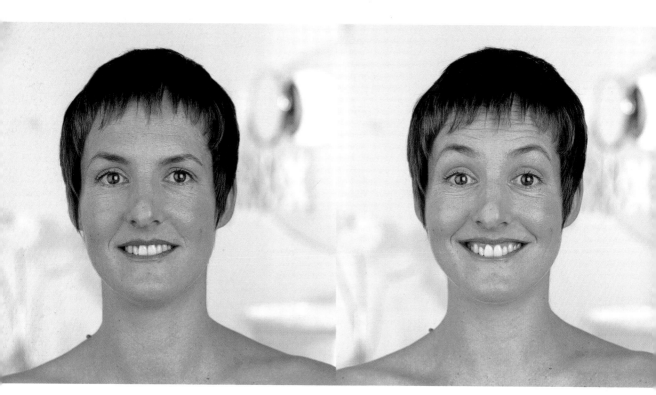

Toning Exercise 6: Neck Tension Exerciser

As we age, the neck loses tone.

To locate the muscles of your neck, tighten your jaw and lower lip muscles, making your lower lip as wide as you can (see below).

- Drop your head back so you are looking towards the ceiling.

- Clench the muscles of the neck and lower lip so that they work to pull your head back down.

- Repeat 5 times.

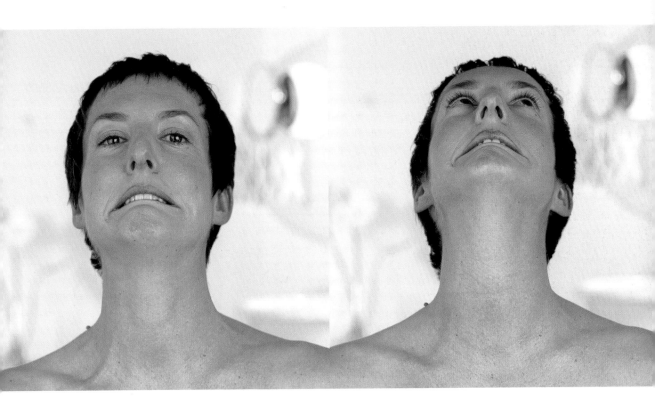

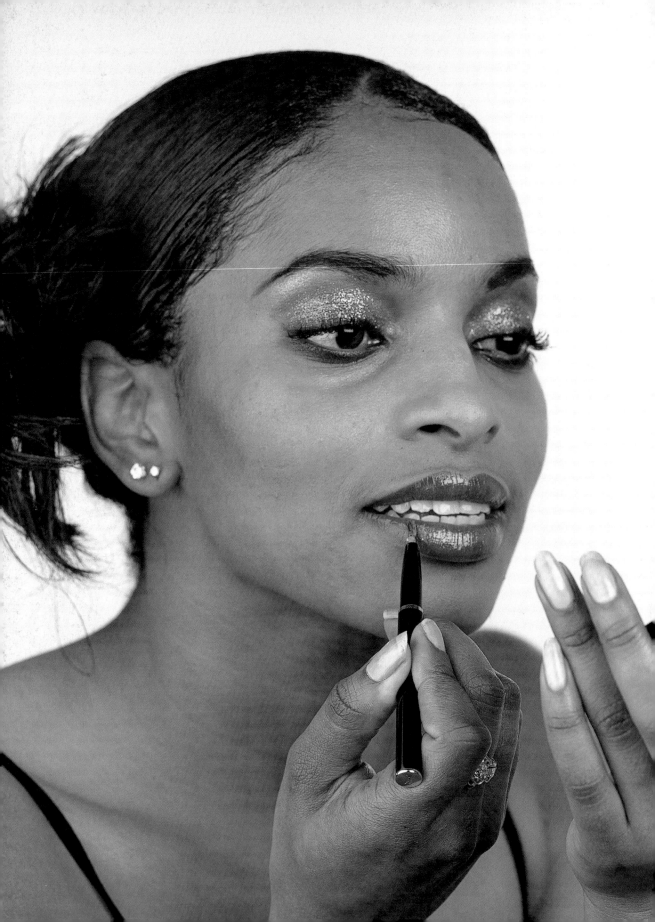

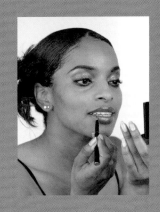

nurture

make-up

Sometimes our faces can benefit from a little more help. The simplest way to give your appearance a lift is to use make-up in a skilful way. I am fortunate in being able to draw on the knowledge of Armand, one of the most talented young make-up artists working in the UK today. He is a master of disguise and here, for the first time, he reveals the approaches used by the professionals for helping to accentuate your best features and down-play your least flattering ones. He also shares the secret-weapon whispers of the stars, and recommends the best cosmetics on the market today, the ones that really do work.

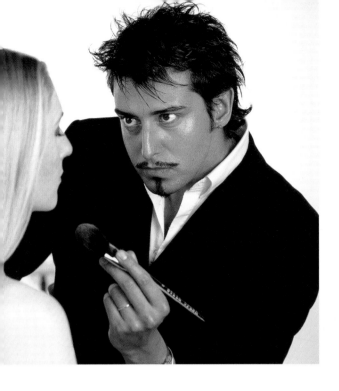

make-up secrets with armand

Without make-up and lipstick, let's face it, we look lacklustre. We can all benefit from the judicious use of some make-up, using it skilfully to enhance what nature has given us. 'Remember, just like clothing, it's not what you wear, but how you wear it,' says Armand. Unfortunately, as with other areas of the beauty industry, cosmetics attract jargon like flies to fly paper. With the help of Armand I am going to cut that out and get down to the essentials, letting you in on the secrets of the professionals, and only telling you what you really need to know.

I first met Armand on GMTV. I am their beauty expert and he is their make-up specialist. Armand excelled in theatrical make-up while training as an actor and dancer. In 1994 he began work with some of the most prestigious cosmetic companies such as Clinique and Yves Saint Laurent before becoming the UK and Eire's make-up artist for the couture house, Givenchy. In September 1998, Armand opened the first personal beauty studio outside London, having familiarized himself, through intense training, with products produced by companies including Sisley, MAC and Estée Lauder. In July 2000, Armand formed his own company, Armand International Ltd, through which he focuses on work within the media. He has worked with celebrities including Claire Sweeney, Tracy Shaw and Sue Johnston, and he's even made-over Anne Widdecombe on GMTV. His work has also appeared in magazines such as *Hello!*, *Vogue*, *Harpers and Queen*, *Marie Claire*, *She* and *OK!* 'You want make-up to look good, not obvious,' he urges.

Actress Tracey Shaw: 'She loves the Sisley Glossy lip gloss because it contains particles which are like multi-colour glitter particles which gives a fuller look to the lips and smells fab. She never goes to a premiere without her La Prairie Extrait de Caviar, which evens her complexion, brightens the skin and ensures make-up stays perfect all night long,' says Armand.

Shobna Gulati (Sunetta in *Coronation Street*): 'She swears by Laura Mercier Crushed Hazelnut Blusher. Because of her skin-tone, it's guaranteed to give her a boost of colour without looking too obvious.'

One world-famous British pop star uses Vaseline on her lips and also mixes it with her foundation to give her skin a glossy finish.

Award-winning actress **Sue Johnston** (of *Brookside* fame, *The Royle Family*, and several motion pictures): 'She likes a fairly smoky look to her eyes. But a heavy look around the eye can make the eyes look smaller, so she opens them with Eyelure Individual Lashes applied to the outer edge of the eye.'

Disguise

Covering Up Age Spots

Be careful not to use products that will clog the skin. Beauty is about enhancing, not masking, your features. But nonetheless, everyone has imperfections that they would prefer to disguise. Fortunately there are some great cover-up foundations and concealers on the market. Dermablend and MAC both have a good range, as do Clinique. Always use concealer after you've applied your foundation. Less is more, so pat sparingly on the affected area before applying powder over the top to set.

Freckles

It's always best not to hide these, first because it's impractical, particularly if you are a redhead, and secondly because these are not imperfections. However much make-up you use they will respond with intensified pigmentation in the sun. The best thing you can do to downplay them is to wear a 35-plus factor sunblock so they do not darken further.

Birthmarks

Apply concealer to affected area after using foundation. If your blemish is very blue or red it's worth investing in the Lancôme Pro Palette, which is designed to disguise imperfections. Use the green shade to tone down red marks, the yellow shade to tone down blue marks.

Spots

Before applying make-up use a skin care product to help dry out the spot. Alternatively, for more radical emergency help invest in Spot Control Formula by Prescriptives, or Anti Blemish Spot Cream by Clinique.

After applying foundation, choose a liquid emollient concealer which will help disguise the spot rather than drawing attention to it with a dryer concealer. You only need a tiny amount applied with a cotton bud rather than your finger (to prevent infection).

Your hormonal cycle means you are bound to get blemishes around your chin at certain times. If they are very raised, angry or red use a bit of the Lancôme Pro Palette green concealer over the top of a skin care treatment, followed by a dab of normal concealer and a dusting of pressed powder. If the spot is very raised, minimize it by using a slightly deeper shade of concealer.

Specs Appeal

If you are short-sighted your eyes will tend to look smaller when wearing prescription lenses. If you are long-sighted, your glasses will tend to magnify your eyes from an observer's point of view.

Short-sightedness

Your short sight at least means you don't have any difficulty seeing clearly to apply make-up! You can flatter your eyes by making them appear larger. Focus some darker shadow at the outer edge of the eye around the eyelashes. Use paler or iridescent shadow towards the inner corner of the eye and as a highlighter under the eyebrows. Mascara is very important here, as it will help open the eyes. A good curling mascara is Helena Rubenstein Vertiginous Mascara, which will make your eyelashes long and luscious.

Long-sightedness

You might find it difficult to focus clearly on the fine close-up detail required to apply make-up. Invest in a magnifying mirror and consider buying glasses with pivoting lenses so you can make up each eye with one lens flicked up. Nothing is so ageing as badly applied make-up, so your tools are essential.

To prevent your eyes looking over-large, apply eyeliner to the inside edge of the skin under the eyes to help reduce their impact a little bit. Choose more muted colours, as glasses magnify the effect and you don't want your eyes to dominate the rest of your face. Use lashings of mascara so your eyes don't appear too closed up.

Choosing Specs

When choosing glasses make sure they have an anti-glare facility on the lens so they don't spoil the look of your eye make-up.

If you have a round face	Choose oblong-style glasses, perhaps slightly wider at the outer edge. This will help give a more angular appearance to your face.
Squarer face	Choose glasses with a softer, slightly curving rim to soften the face.
Oval face	Choose a softer-shaped frame in a longer, wide oval shape to give definition.
Triangular face	You should choose fairly narrow frames so you don't over-emphasize the wider part of your face.

Large lenses are currently very fashionable, but they are not timeless. If you do choose them, opt for a pair which are frameless, as these are far more flattering for the eye.

breakout: clever colour

Changing Your Face Shape

Although there are many different face shapes, some people feel conscious that their own appearance is in need of a bit of cosmetic enhancement. Fortunately you do not have to involve an expensive surgeon in order to make subtle changes. The key is using variations in the colour of bronzers, blushers and powders either to minimize over-strong features or to accentuate weaker areas of your face using the principle of shading. Your face is a blank canvas on which you can use colour to create an illusion.

Blending is the key to a natural look. Choose a shade of foundation that is the same as the skin tone of your neck, and manipulate it by layering over powders and bronzers with good-quality brushes. Remember: Darkness recedes and lightness enhances. Foundation oxidizes and can turn a slightly darker shade half an hour after application.

These techniques are all especially useful at night-time when lighting is less harsh. Be more subtle in the daytime.

For a Round Face

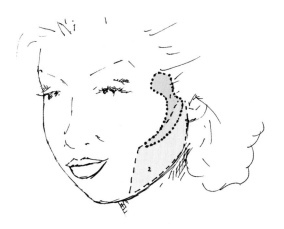

1 Use blusher or bronzer to create the appearance of a hollow in the side of the cheek. Smile, then brush the colour just under the fleshy part of the cheek, following the jaw line.

2 Alternatively, use a slightly deeper shade of foundation underneath the cheekbone blending around the jawline – this will take the edge off the roundness and create a more sculptured contour.

Avoid using glossy products on the skin because these can give added fullness to the face, especially on the cheekbones.

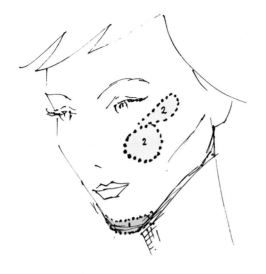

For a Triangular Face

1 Use a darker shade around the chin area to blunt the chin.

2 Applying paler powder or highlighter on the cheekbones, as well as a dab onto the fleshy part of the cheek, will allow light to flatter your face while drawing attention away from your chin, giving a fuller look to those areas.

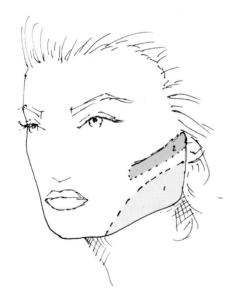

For a Square Strong-jawed Face

1 Focus your attention on the edge of the jawline towards the ear, and apply a deeper shade over this area. This will appear to soften and remove the angularity of your jaw.

2 You should also emphasize your cheekbones with a sharp line drawn underneath them in a deeper shade of powder or bronzer. Carefully blend it in to play up a more hollowed look that will both balance the strength of your jaw and draw attention away from it.

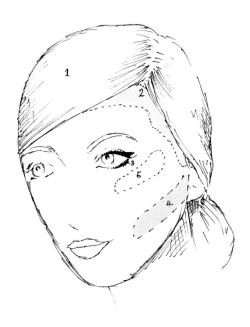

For an Oval-shaped Face

1 People with oval faces tend to have quite high foreheads. First of all you need to choose a hairstyle that sweeps the hair onto the forehead.

2 Then, use a slightly deeper shade of powder to minimize the forehead's impact.

3 If your eyes are not particularly large, emphasize them using eyeliner on the edges of the eye.

4 You should also sculpt the cheekbones by defining underneath with deeper powder and just a little bit of gloss on the cheekbone.

Thin Lips

To give the illusion of a fuller look, try using foundation over your lips as well as the rest of your face. Then shade in the outer edges with a pale or neutral lip liner, avoiding a dark pencil which will make your lips look smaller. Leave the central fleshy part bare before applying a lip gloss to give a moist, pouty look.

The trouble with many lip glosses is that they are easily licked away, so try Diorific Plastic Shine by Christian Dior, or Make Up For Ever gloss, both of which have improved staying power.

I would strongly recommend that anyone with thin lips uses lip gloss which helps thin lips to look fuller and more three-dimensional. Various products have been devised specifically to help create the illusion of bigger, plumper lips without resorting to surgery.

Lip Plump by BeneFit works on the idea that your lips need a foundation as well. Using a combination of liquid waxes, it builds up a layer on the lip which fills the fine lines of the lip and, when dry, provides a fuller, plumper lip on which to apply lip liner and lipstick.

Lip liners are useful because they prevent lipstick bleeding or creeping up the fine lines that surround our mouths as we age. It also looks much more polished by enhancing our natural lip line, which is often blurred by wearing lipstick alone.

Radiant Touch by Yves Saint Laurent is a handy little highlighter pen that can be used all around the periphery of the lips, just beyond the lip line. It brightens skin once it has been blended in and creates the effect of fuller-looking lips when light hits that area. It contains self-adapting pigments, so one shade suits all, but be aware that a little goes a long way – don't overdo it. You should then use lip liner in the usual way and fill in with lipstick or gloss.

Large Nose

Skilful use of powder, using slight changes in colour, is the way to decrease the impact of a larger nose. Never use bronzer here – your T-zone produces a lot of oil, and only powder can absorb it as well as offering a more subtle pigment than that found in a bronzer.

If you have a wide nose, use a slightly deeper shade on either side of the bridge of the nose, avoiding the bridge itself. This will appear to slim it.

If you have a prominent Roman hook, draw a slightly deeper shade of powder down the centre of your nose. You should also apply highlighter to your cheekbones and accentuate your eyes to help balance your strong nose. Also use a small amount under the tip of the nose to take away the sharpness.

Over-hanging Lids

This is often a symptom of ageing, but it can easily be overcome. To find out if your lids are beginning to droop, look dead straight into your mirror – if your eyelid appears to be covered by a fold of skin from your brow bone, your lids are over-hanging.

Where the skin touches the lashes give a touch of colour, just as if it were an eyelid. Next, raise your eyebrows so that the skin is taut, and tilt your head up. Blend in the colour you've applied so that it is not a stark stripe. Blending is key. When you relax your face back you'll still have a haze of colour, and when you express yourself and your eyes rise you won't see an obvious stripe of colour.

You should use the same principle if you are Oriental, with the addition of liquid liner applied next to the top set of lashes to accentuate the shape of your eye.

If you find that eyeshadow creases, use an eye shadow base. Clinique makes a good one, and MAC's Fast Response Eye Cream will help firm up the area. If you want to treat yourself, splash out on Protective Eye Base by Guerlain, which is a blend of waxes which clings on to colour and is the best of the lot.

Chin Reductions

Using a slightly deeper tone of powder or bronzer around the chin area will help to diminish the impact of your chin (also see 'Changing Your Face Shape: For a Triangular Face', above).

If you have a chin that drops away into your neck, whether a double chin or the beginnings of a double chin, you can create a jawline for yourself using make-up. Make sure you use a touch-resistant foundation or powder so your newly enhanced chin doesn't brush off onto your collar! Lift your chin up and brush powder one to two shades darker than your own skin tone from the jawline down to the Adam's apple (yes, women have one, though it's smaller because their vocal cords are smaller than men's). This really does give a more sculptured look to the jaw, and sets the face apart from the neck.

How to Choose Colour for Your Skin

Finding a make-up that flatters you is a great way to look fresh and polished. But don't be fearful about experimenting. It's not brain surgery, it's make-up, and you should always treat it as fun. There are lots of cheap and cheerful colours available, but it is definitely worth spending a bit more. The colours will last longer and you will be able to blend them together. Also be aware that make-up will look different in different lights. Always try out your look under two different light sources – for example, bathroom and next to a window – otherwise the results could be scary.

Always make up in the following sequence, which will help you control the effect you are creating:

1 Foundation (creates a canvas)
2 Eyes (the focus of your look)
3 Lips (to balance the eyes)
4 Cheeks (to complete and balance the whole look).

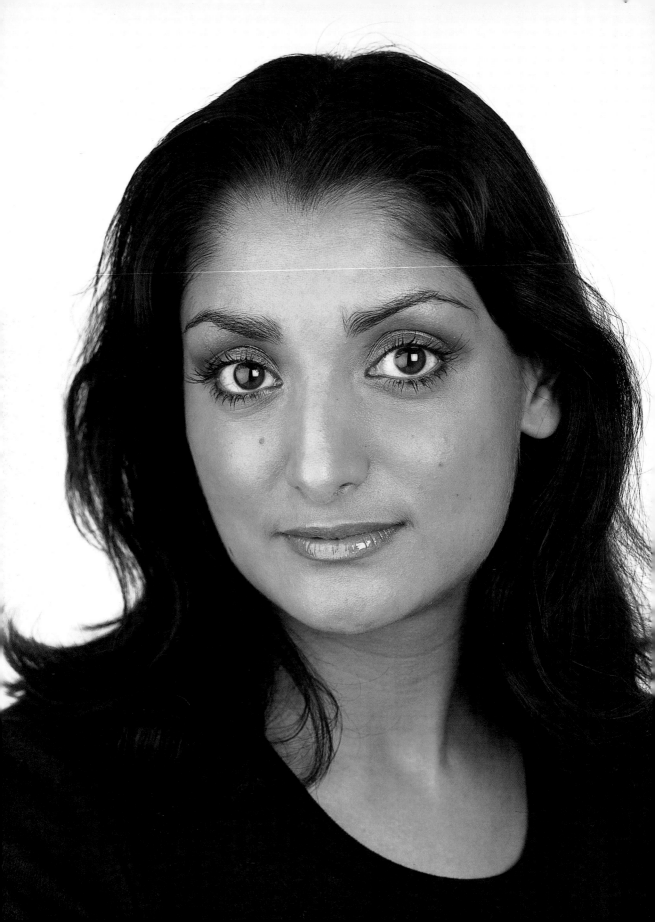

Raj

Beauty Role Model: Marie Helvin, Penelope Cruz

Thoughts about make-up: I always wear make-up and wouldn't leave the house without it. But I've never had the nerve to experiment with false lashes – I feel they'd look too 'fake'.

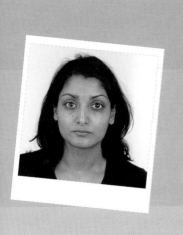

Skin
Foundation: Dermacolour D5 by Dermablend
Cover Up: Palette Pro by Lancôme

Eyes
Shadow: Gold and Brown by Shu Uemura
Glitter: Gold by Mac
Line:
Mascara: Extra Superlash by Rimmel
Lashes: Individual false lashes by Eyeline

Lips
Line:
Colour: Glacé Shimmer by Shu Uemura

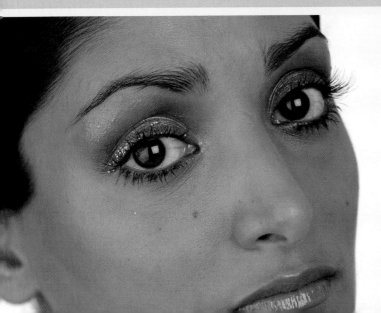

Choosing Foundation

The best approach to choosing a foundation that flatters your skin tone is to try the foundations on your jaw-line. Pick three shades close to your skin tone – the one that appears to disappear into your skin is the one that is perfect for you. Make sure you check the colour in natural light before buying. Using the jaw is the best way to match the colour to your neck tone (never use the inside of your wrist, as this is far paler than either neck or jaw). Generally, our faces are uneven in tone – some areas are red, others blue, others ruddy. Foundation is there to perfect the complexion, to even out these variations, not to mask the skin. So only apply foundation to the areas that need it. Always blend the colour out thoroughly so that the skin on your jaw has no foundation.

If you are not confident you've found the perfect shade, or have problem skin, it's worth investing in a custom-made blend. Both Prescriptives and Elizabeth Arden have an in-store service – for approximately £25 you receive a consultation and a customized foundation. You can also decide on the consistency or coverage rate.

Choosing Eye Colour

I have always maintained that anybody can wear any colour, it just boils down to the 'B' word – Blending. But if you want to play safe, here are a few ideas:

Blue eyes	Choose gold, russet or brown tones to enhance the colour of your eyes. Don't use blue eye shadow, it will reduce the intensity of your natural blue pigment.
Green eyes	Lilac is extremely flattering.
Hazel eyes	Warm tones such as amber, terracotta, taupe and brick brown will bring out the tones in the eye, but avoid flat browns, which will make you look tired.
Dark brown eyes	Shades of blue, grey and silver are flattering, but keep it light to bring out tones within the eye effectively.
Red heads	You are likely to have a fairly pink tone to your skin, so avoid using pink colours around your eye area as they will make your eyes look sore. Instead, go for brown or green tones.

Choosing Lip Colour

You can have a free hand. If you like it, then it's working. The most effective way to assess a colour is to dab it on your fingertip and hold it against your face to see its impact.

Turning Up the Volume for Make-up on the Move

If you tend to wear a minimal amount of make-up during the day – perhaps just mascara and lipstick – here's a quick method to turn up the volume for the evening which doesn't involve carting loads of different products around.

Draw brown eye-liner across the outer edge of your upper eye lid, close to the lashes, and smudge it in. For a stronger look apply another smudge to the lower eyelash at the outer edge of the eye, moving inwards and fading to nothing. Use the eyeliner in your eyebrows as well, and smudge in to intensify the brow. Be subtle and refer to your natural brow colour. Put on another coat of mascara (upper lashes only). Use clear gloss at the centre of lips to give a hint of a pout.

Simone

Beauty Role Model: Aaliyah – had the same skin tones and colour mix

Thoughts about make-up: I wear lots of browns, golds and bronzes to compliment my skin tones, but I'm never sure how to dress this up to go from 'day to night'.

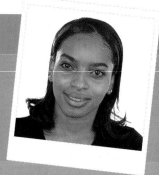

Look 1 Daywear		Look 2 Dressed Up	
Skin		**Skin**	
Foundation:	Dermablend	Foundation:	
Cover Up:		Cover Up:	
Blush:	Drive Me Jelly by Helena Rubenstein	Blush:	
Eyes		**Eyes**	
Shadow:	Love in the Mist by Vincent Longo	Shadow:	Valerian by Alchemy
		Glitter:	Gold by Make Up For Ever
Line:	Liquid liner in Black by Shu Uemura	Line:	
Mascara:	Extencils by Lancôme	Mascara:	Magnificils by Lancôme
Lips		**Lips**	
Line:	Nude by Bobbi Brown	Line:	Raisin by Bobbi Brown
Colour:	Sheer Transparent # 9 by Giorgio Armani	Colour:	Nico by Mac

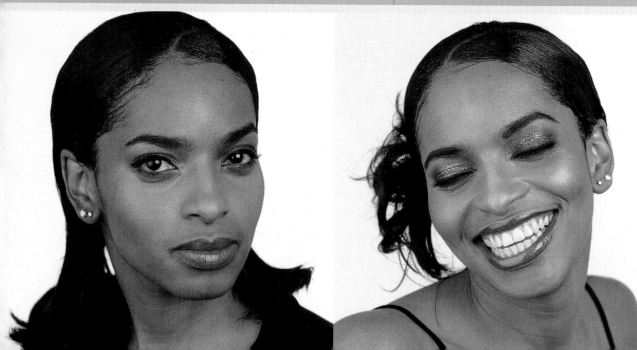

Make-up for Brows

Fill in any blank spots with eyebrow pencil or powder in a colour a shade lighter than your own eyebrow hair. The result will be a totally natural-looking brow. Pencil is good for darkening or defining brows without adding volume; use it to draw in individual hairs or to strengthen the brow for a more definite look. Powder is good for adding volume and filling in a sparse brow.

Givenchy eyebrow pencil in blonde is good for most skin tones. It is a taupe brown that is easy to blend into the natural brow without looking obvious.

If you have dark skin choose Browzing by BeneFit, it's a coloured wax in four different shades that is soft and easy to apply for a polished look.

make-up for ageing skin

Foundation

Wearing foundation with wrinkles helps to reduce their visual impact, but only if you choose the right product. You need to select a liquid foundation to help hydrate the skin. Compact foundations tend to emphasize lined skin because they are very drying. But some liquid foundations can be too heavy. You want something that gives coverage without looking plastered. My recommendation for mature skin is Yves Saint Laurent Line Smoothing Foundation.

However, if you are a die-hard user of compact foundation, try Hydra Compact Foundation by Lancôme. It's one of the few compact foundations which look good with more mature skin, it has good coverage and offers staying power.

Whatever foundation you choose, make sure you blend it out to the jawline.

If prone to age spots or liver spots, use concealer after foundation but before applying powder.

Eyes

Avoid using pearlized or iridescent eye shadow at the outer edge of the eye, where fine lines are more likely. Wear them instead towards the inner edge of the eye, or as a highlighter under the eyebrow. Choose matt shadow at the edges – matt shadows are finely milled and less likely to accentuate lines.

Laughter Lines

Use Yves Saint Laurent Radiant Touch brightener, which appears to minimize lines because of the way the product catches the light and bounces it back, creating an optical illusion.

Lips

Use lip liner to stop lipstick 'bleeding' up the tiny lines that tend to surround the mouth with age. With age all lips tend to recede and lose some of their plumpness – use a dab of gloss in the centre of the lips to help imply a natural pout.

Dull Skin

An expensive approach – but one to consider before resorting to a face lift – is applying one of the specialist youth flashes, also known as make-up primers, that are available from department stores. These are serums applied under make-up which lift and smooth mature skin and help to give it a warm, youthful glow.

These are my tips for the most effective. At the more affordable end of the scale is Beauty Flash Balm by Clarins. More expensive is Tensor Immediate Lift by Sisley, which is a serum you apply twice a week under foundation. The best, and more expensive, product for that no-holds-barred approach is Caviar for the Face by La Prairie. It contains Iranian Beluga caviar, which is one the brightest substances in use in a cosmetic. It will emerge through your make-up and give your face a delicious luminescence, as well as a firming feeling.

armand's guide to the cosmetic jargon jungle

Accent	Simply, to accentuate a part of the face such as the cheekbones
Allergy-tested	All ingredients have been monitored for reaction by patch tests conducted on selected volunteers or skin cultures over a period of time (compare with hypoallergenic)
Apple of the cheeks	The fleshy part which emerges when we smile
Bronzer	A product designed to give a sun-kissed look anywhere on the body. Can be used alongside or on top of blusher (used to give colour rather than the illusion of a suntan).
Contour of the eye	A fancy way of referring to the eye socket
Hypoallergenic	All known major allergic ingredients have been removed (compare with allergy-tested)
Light-diffusing	A luminescent effect in some make-up achieved by adding microscopically small particles that filter the light in all directions. Often used in foundations where they help to emphasize contours.
Light-reflecting	An effect produced in some make-up that gives a mirror-like brightness, particularly when viewed straight on. Often used in concealers where it helps to hide dark circles and blemishes.
Matt	Flat, non-light-reflecting
Microspheres	Cosmetic-speak for particularly tiny particles of make-up that allow the make-up to follow the contours of the skin more closely and penetrate more effectively between the dead cells of the upper layers
Non-comedogenic	A cosmetic designed so that pores won't be blocked. Particularly appropriate for acne sufferers.
Opthamologically-tested	A product that has been tested as being eye safe
Sheer	Minimal coverage
Undertone	This is the colour running underneath your actual skin colour, which you want to counterbalance or even out with foundation or concealer. Extremes are a blue undertone in a black skin, a red undertone in a

	red-head, or a yellow undertone (also known as a sallow complexion) in an Asian skin.
Water-proof	Contains an ingredient that acts as a water barrier and means make-up is suitable for use in the pool or on the beach
Water-resistant	Contains an ingredient to make the cosmetic adhere to the skin and act as a barrier to moisture. Usually means tear-resistant – you can cry in it, but not swim in it. Efficacy will reduce over time.

armand's top ten professional insights

1. Hangover Pencil

Invest in an eye brightener from Lancôme or Guerlain. These are white pencils with a hint of green that are brilliant for damage limitation. Run the pencil along the lower lid, just inside the eye, to neutralize any redness and make your eyes appear to sparkle.

2. Shadow Blotter

Before applying eye-shadow, dust loose translucent powder underneath the eye, enabling you to brush away any spillage after you've finished making up your eyes.

3. The Perfect Pout

Apply foundation on the lips, followed by lipstick. Blot with one ply of tissue, then, with the tissue still in place, dust loose powder over the top. A fine mist of powder will diffuse through the thin tissue and set your lipstick.

4. Clever Lips

To prevent transferring lipstick onto your glass or cup, wet your finger and run it around the rim.

5. Lip Care

If you suffer with flaky lips, especially in the winter, brush your lips with a baby toothbrush and apply Kiehls Lip Balm or Lip Saver by Molton Brown.

6. Back-comb Your Lashes

To help make your eyelashes look longer, apply a coat of mascara on the top side of the upper lashes – this will mop up any excess eye shadow. Then apply another coat on the underside of the lashes from root to tip in a zig zag motion to make them look thicker.

7. Glamour Lashes

Treat yourself to a couple of Eyelure Individual Lashes and glue them onto the outer corner to give instant glamour and a wider-eyed look.

8. Best Application Brush

The most sensational piece of kit on the market is the Bobbi Brown Bluepoint Squirrel brush, the ultimate way to apply loose powder. Because the brush tapers to a point you can direct powder right up under the eyes with no smudging.

9. Healthy Nails

For strong, good-looking finger armour, munch on one jelly cube a day.

10. And Finally ...

Remember, your make-up is only as good as your skin. Make-up is no substitute for good skin care.

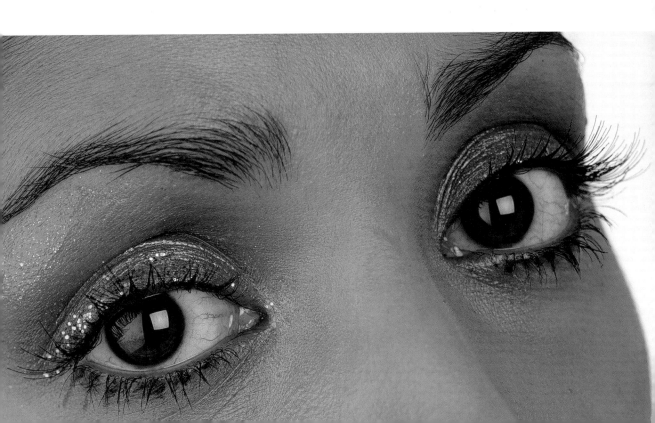

natural make-up tips

Natural-looking make-up is one of the toughest of all looks to achieve. Think about it: you want to look as if you've got fantastic skin and yet wear hardly any make-up. Very few people have fantastic skin, so you can see why this is a challenge. The key here is preparation, and the watchword is 'detail'.

Eyebrows are very important to this polished look. The less make-up you wear, the more your eyebrows exert an influence on the overall look. Eyebrow shape is critical (see Make-up for Brows, page 141). Once shaped perfectly with all strays removed, apply Mr Mascara Brow Gel or Christian Dior Brow Gel to smooth them perfectly into position.

Apply three coats of black/brown mascara or clear mascara.

Concealer is very important under the eyes, where you want to remove any sign of redness or bagginess. One of the best products to use is M&S Perfect Concealer, which has a sun protection factor of 15. Choose a tone that is slightly lighter than your natural skin tone around the eye, and apply in the indentation close to the nose in a series of tiny dots smudged in with your ring finger, which minimizes pressure on the skin.

To make your eyes look wider and brighter, apply a tiny dot of Radiant Touch (Yves Saint Laurent) at the outer corner, where fine lines tend to develop, and smudge it in. Apply another couple of tiny dots on the laughter lines by the side of the nose, and smudge in.

Finally, to give a sun-kissed look to your 'un-made up' face, use a little bit of bronzer where you would naturally tan – on the forehead, down the nose, on the cheekbones and T-zone – but remember that less is more.

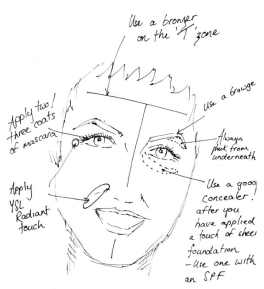

Use a bronzer on the 'T' zone

Apply two / three coats of mascara

Use a brow gel

Always pluck from underneath

Apply YSL Radiant touch

Use a good concealer! after you have applied a touch of sheer foundation – use one with an SPF

Stella

Beauty Role Model: No one in particular

Thoughts about make-up: I don't wear make-up at all – it's just not important to me.

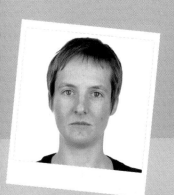

Skin
Foundation: Warm 2 by Marks & Spencer
Cover Up: Lucidity in Very Light by Estée Lauder
Corrector: Palette Pro 01 by Lancôme
Powder: Diffusing Powder by Alchemy

Eyes
Shadow:
Line:
Mascara: Lash Discovery One by One by Maybelline
Line:
Mascara: Lash Discovery One by One by Maybelline
Brows: Blonde by Givenchy

Lips
Line: Spice by Mac
Colour: Gloss 01 by Make Up For Ever

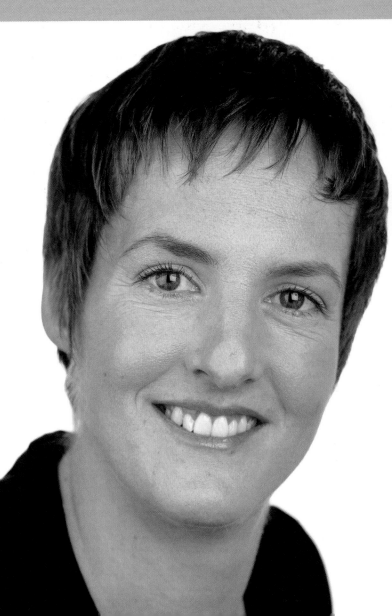

Tips for the Different Skin Types

Oily

Use oil-free products for the face. If you have acne-prone skin, choose a medicated foundation. Use a pressed powder on the T-zone to absorb excess oil, such as MAC's Studio Finish Powder which is very matt but doesn't look thick or cakey. Try using compact rather than liquid foundation, but if you prefer to use liquid then try Superfit Foundation by Clinique, which is water-resistant, long-wearing, completely oil-free and comes in a wide range of shades. Around the eye area use an eye base to prevent creasing of the eye shadow. For any blemishes use Crème Camphrea by Guerlain, which is medicated and tinted, and also contains zinc which is known for its beneficial properties to the skin.

Open Pores

If you suffer from open pores, Pore Minimizing Make-up by Clinique is excellent. It's a mix of oil and foundation that you shake into an emulsion before use.

Dry Skin

This tends to be prone to flakiness; your starting point should be good skin care with a particular emphasis on polishing to remove any loose flaky skin (see page 17). Choose a fluid, rather than compact, foundation. My recommendations are Givenchy Cream Foundation or Estée Lauder's Double Wear, both of which help to gently moisturize the skin. You could also try Hydrating Foundation by Marks & Spencer. If you need to use powder, choose a loose rather than pressed one and apply it to the tip of your nose to avoid it looking flaky. Avoid using powder blushers which can dry the skin; a good cream blush which will be more comfortable on the skin is Nars The Multiple which is an emollient cream stick you can use on your eyes, cheeks and lips. Similarly, Christian Dior's The Multi-Touch and Benefit 911 can be used on all areas. In all cases your skin will appreciate the moistness of the product.

Combination Skin

If you have combination skin, use oil-based products on your cheeks and more drying products on the T-zone.

Dull Skin

Good skin care is the key to brightening your complexion, yet some foundations can be relied on to give you a quick-fix 'healthy glow'. Try Helena Rubenstein's Illumination Foundation which, because of its 'light-modulator', proves invaluable on skin with uneven pigmentation. This is a patented ingredient which appears to scatter light over the skin.

The Importance of the Right Foundation

Foundation shouldn't clog or be cakey, but should work in harmony with your skin, enhancing, not masking your features. You want people to comment on how fantastic your skin is, not how great your foundation looks. Women don't need the sort of full-on coverage that was fashionable in the past. In the eighties it was worn heavily, before becoming more natural in the nineties. Women are now more in control of their lives and are rediscovering their femininity, so slapping on foundation has become redundant. Use foundation only to enhance your looks, and never trowel it on. Everyone should opt for light-to-medium coverage, using medium-to-heavy formulations only where you need it and blending it out to your own skin tone.

It's definitely worth spending a bit more to buy a product that performs. The more expensive ones look like skin, not like foundation. Your foundation is not just make-up, it should also be part of your skin care regime, so make sure it contains a sun protection factor to protect you from both infra red and UVA rays.

Use your fingers to manipulate and apply foundation, as you'll have much better control. Dab it on to the back of your hand first, like an artist's palette. This will also melt the product and make it more pliable.

Jean

Beauty Role Model: Nicole Kidman

Thoughts about make-up: I only wear very light make-up usually. I'm quite conscious of having red cheeks but I'm not sure how to cover this up without looking a bit 'caked'. I'm getting married soon and there will be a lot of lilac and purple in the colour scheme so I would like to see if I can carry off these colours.

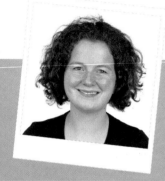

Skin
Foundation: 01 by Prescriptives
Cover Up: Radiant Touch by Yves Saint Laurent
Powder: Beige by Shu Uemura

Eyes
Shadow: Lavender Mist by Vincent Longo
Line:
Mascara: Vertiginous Brown Spectacular by Helena Rubenstein

Lips
Line: Noisette by Shu Uemura
Colour: Apricot Glaze by Stila

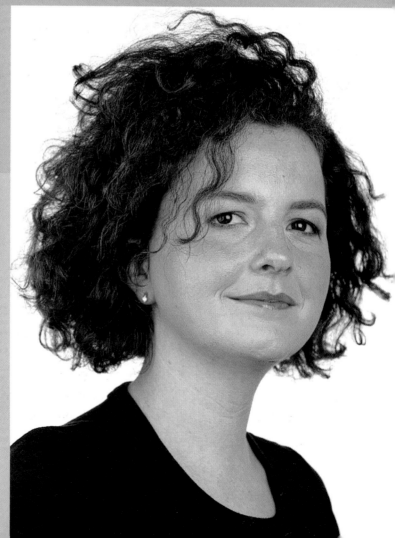

Tricks to Help Your Make-up Last All Day

Use a make-up primer underneath your foundation to help make-up stay in place.

If you want your make-up to stay put with the minimum of touch-ups, avoid using shiny or glossy products anywhere near the T-zone.

To give your cheekbones an enduring dewy look, use Elizabeth Arden's Eight-Hour Cream on the cheekbone, or Emporio Armani's Shimmering Fluid foundation. Avoid using glossy products such as these anywhere near the oil-generating areas of the face.

There are many lip stains and sticks sold as kiss-proof, but I recommend these for good all-day-long endurance:

Lipfinity by Max Factor is exceptionally good. It's a two-part system that comes with a clear balm applied before the lipstick.

Extrait de Rouge by Chanel and Rouge Magnetique by Lancôme both have good staying power.

Lipcote is a sealer applied over your own lipstick which is effective if you want a glossy finish. Some long-lasting lip colours can be drying, so make sure your lips are well-moisturized and prepared beforehand.

Keep your compact powder close to hand to pat skin dry every few hours.

Avoid using mascara on the bottom lashes, which is in any case considered passé. Not only will they look like spider's legs, but over the course of the day the mascara will undoubtedly end up on your cheek. For a more enduring lower lash-lengthening approach, use a touch of shadow underneath the lower outer corner.

If you are going somewhere hot or humid, such as a night-club or tropical holiday, consider using a make-up fixer. Origins Sprinkler System is a hydration system with orange blossom, coriander and coconut oil which acts as a fixer and instant hydrator. A cheaper approach is to use a squirt of fine mist hair spray, such as Elnette. Make sure you give your skin a patch test first. Ensuring your eyes are shut, it is important to hold the canister at arm's reach and spray in the swiftest of bursts towards your face. Alternatively, spray into the air in front of you and waft your face through the particles as they fall (this is also a good tip for scenting your hair with perfume).

For tips on how to stop lipstick running, see page 144.

The Truth About Applying Blusher

Apply blusher last. Once your eyes and lips are made up you'll know how much you need to carry off the look. Blusher has two effects: it helps to define your facial structure by highlighting the cheekbones, and it also gives warmth to the skin, particularly when you are using a foundation.

Blending in your blusher, be it cream or compact, is the main key, and it's worth investing in a good brush. Blusher must always look natural.

Build blusher up gradually. First of all, smile to locate the 'apple' of your cheek. Start off with a dab of blusher on the apple and blend upwards towards your temple. Do the same on the other side. Stand back and take a look at the whole picture, which will inform you whether you need to apply a little more, or to remove a little colour.

Skin tone influences the colour you should choose. Bronzers are good for sculptural definition rather than colour, but if you do use a bronzer it's a good idea to put just a dab of colour onto the apple of your cheeks to introduce a bit of natural warmth:

If you have warmer tones (brown hair, more olive skin)	Use a peachy tone on the apple of your cheeks
If you have fairer tones (blonde hair, paler skin)	Use a little dab of pink on the cheeks
If you have black or Asian skin	Use a russet tone on the cheeks

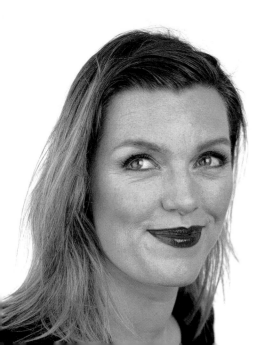

label-watching

You may not have the time or inclination to make your own cosmetic treatments. If you opt for shop-bought, take time to read labels carefully. Try to choose products with natural ingredients where possible, and if you have sensitive skin choose hypo-allergenic products. But bear in mind that although 42 per cent of women believe they have sensitive skin, according to a recent study many of them are suffering from irritation caused by chemicals in the skin-care products they use. This is not to say that every woman will react badly, but your chances of a bad reaction are increased if you choose to use products containing the ingredients listed below.

The main culprits are the colour and fragrance chemicals, but preservatives and UV absorbers can also play a part. Adverse reactions from chemicals in skin-care products include allergies and dermatitis.

If you don't like the idea of putting petrochemicals and high concentrations of preservative (often formaldehyde-based) onto your skin, shop around for vegetable-based ranges. But read the small print. Many so-called 'natural' products contain only a tiny amount of plant extract.

Do try and avoid the products mentioned below, which can be damaging to your skin.

FD&C or D&C followed by a colour reference number	These are synthetic colours which are potentially carcinogenic, and should be avoided at all costs
Hydroxycitronellal	This has been linked to psoriasis
Linalool (or Linalol)	This has been linked to psoriasis
Mono-, di- and triethanolamine	Common thickening agents used in cleansers that can lead to skin dryness and interfere with hormones
Parabens (ethyl-parabens, methyl-parabens, propyl-parabens, butyl-parabens)	Preservatives that can cause skin rashes and allergic reactions

Perfumes	Most perfumes contain petrochemicals, which penetrate the skin and may cause toxic reactions, headaches, skin irritations and dizziness
Petrolatum (or mineral oil)	This is a bulking agent made from low-grade petroleum oil, which has no nutritional value, strips away the skin's own natural oils leading to dry skin conditions, and can cause the skin to become over-sensitive to sunlight
Propylene glycol	A key ingredient in antifreeze, made from petrochemicals or from alcohol mixed with glycerine, which can cause toxic and allergic reactions
Sodium Lauryl Sulphate	A chemical degreasing compound often used in foaming cleansers which can lead to allergic reactions and skin rashes

The following ingredients have been linked to **eczema:**

1,2-Dibromo-2,4-dicyanobutane	Methyl Alcohol
Alcohol	Methyldibromo Glutaronitrile
Alcohol denat.	Potassium Tallowate
Butadiene/Acrylonitrile Copolymer	Sodium Lauryl Sulfate
Diammonium	Sodium Tallowate
Dithiodiglycolate	Styrene/Acrylates/Acrylonitrile
Glycol	Copolymer.

The following ingredients are among nearly 300 that have been linked to **dermatitis:**

2-Bromo-2-nitropopane-1,3-diol	Glycolic Acid
Alcohol	Imidazolidinyl Urea
Ammonium Glycolate	Lanolin
Benzyl Alcohol	Oxybenzone
BHA	Sorbitan Palmitate
BHT	Sorbitan Sesquioleate
Cetearyl Alcohol	Stearyl Alcohol
Cetyl Alcohol	t-Butyl Hydroquinone
Choloacetaminde	TEA-Cocoyl
Cocamide DEA, MEA and MIPA	

The following are suspected acne-promoting ingredients and should be avoided if you suffer from **blackheads** or **acne:**

Butyl Stearate	Oleic Acid
Coal Tar	Potassium Tallowate
Decyl Oleate	Propyleneglycol-2-myristyl
Isocetyl Stearate	Propionate
Isolpropyl Isostearate	Sodium Tallowate
Methyl Oleate	Tehobroma Cacao
Myristyl Propionate	Xanthene
Octyl Stearate	Zea Mays

clinic treatments

For some people a more intensive salon treatment might be a consideration. I do not believe in major cosmetic surgery, which so often eradicates personality in the pursuit of perfection. In my opinion, the perfect way to mature is to allow your skin to age naturally while caring for it simply and sensibly. Yet one woman in three toys with the idea of having major aesthetic surgery in Britain, and a recent study by a high-street bank found that one in five loans is used for major cosmetic work.

Instead, I believe in non-invasive salon treatments, such as those offered at my clinic in London, as well as some other out-patient procedures which I only recommend in extreme cases. Here I include a guide so you can educate yourself in the most appropriate treatments for you. Sometimes our faces need more assistance than we can give them with a healthy skin care routine at home, and minor cosmetic surgery on an out-patient basis from a qualified therapist may be appropriate. I only endorse cosmetic surgery in cases where your confidence cannot be lifted by other means. If you've got deep acne or chicken pox scars, for example, or if you have developed deep lines or wrinkles that define the way you look without representing how you feel, then you may be an appropriate candidate. In my clinic I offer only the most natural approaches, but I have decided to include an appraisal of other minor treatments where the emphasis is on beauty rather than intensive surgery, to allow you to best consider the options before committing yourself.

botox

Botox injections, consisting of tiny amounts of botulism toxin, paralyse small facial muscles and are particularly effective on frown lines and crow's feet. The results may take up to 21 days to show, but the injections, which cost approximately £200, are effective for up to six months. When injected in the forehead and eye area, botox prevents patients from frowning or squinting, which protects against progressive worsening of lines and wrinkles.

'I have always been very self-conscious about frowning, I can remember when I was 18 being made aware that I appeared to be scowling all the time. I had my first injection one Christmas, and the difference was amazing. I looked much more relaxed and approachable. It's expensive, but two treatments a year seems a small price to pay for being so much happier with what I see in the mirror.'

Sarah, 39

collagen instant therapy

This is the original 'natural' wrinkle-filler. Introduced in the late 1970s, injectable bovine collagen (made from supporting connective tissue) is still the favourite among many surgeons. The appeal of collagen is that it is versatile, safe and easy to use – but it's not much fun. Like a sewing machine running down a seam, every wrinkle or crow's foot is subjected to multiple punctures, but the small needles make the pinpricks tolerable and you can go straight back to work. Although it is considered safe for 97 per cent of women with wrinkles, a patch test should be offered prior to treatment.

Unfortunately, collagen dissolves after two to four months. It can also lead to temporary bruising and swelling. Costs £200 to £400 per treatment.

mayo-lift

This is a facial-electrolifting treatment that uses a combination of electrical waves and radio frequencies to prevent, correct and arrest the process of facial skin ageing, help reshape and tone muscles, refine wrinkles by acting on muscular, connective and epidermic tissue, and remove trapped toxic build-up from the smaller muscles in the face. It's a face-lift in a box which involves no scarring and is an alternative to surgical lifting.

This is very effective on small and medium-sized wrinkles on the forehead and around the mouth. A special disposable needle is inserted about half a millimetre under the skin's surface in the base of the wrinkle channel. The treatment is not painful and requires no anaesthetic. A pedal is depressed to emit a special radio frequency current for a short burst before the needle is withdrawn. This stimulates the dermis and encourages new cells to form, as well as increasing the elasticity of the skin. Each wrinkle may be treated with two or three emissions in the same session, and will also benefit from micro-dermabrasion (see page 163) to enhance the effect.

Used on a different setting, the machine can also be used to help tighten up sagging cheeks and bags under the eyes, and minimize cellulite and a double chin.

Treatment is not possible if you have a dental prosthesis which could transmit electrical current, if you wear a pacemaker or if you have inflamed skin.

'I'd tried dieting to reduce my double chin, I was so fed up with the large pad of fat that had accumulated there. But nothing seemed to make a difference and my beauty therapist explained that double chins are notoriously difficult areas from which to lose weight. I was told that my two options were surgery or mayo-lift. As I didn't have the money for an operation I decided to try the non-surgical approach. Pairs of tiny needles were pressed sideways into the skin under my jaw line, the skin was kept slightly stretched while they were put in and I could barely feel anything, as they are thinner than a hair, just a mild prick. I'm quite squeamish but it was bearable. There was a fizzy feeling around my jaw as the treatment began that was ticklish, but I soon got used to it. The treatment took between 30 and 40 minutes every fortnight. After the first session I couldn't see any difference, but after the third session my double chin definitely seemed to have reduced in size. After six sessions people started telling me how good I looked and the double chin, although still there, seemed a lot smaller and firmer.'

Sandra, 55

eyelash perm

This treatment, originating from the Far East, is used to curl lashes to help accentuate the eyes and is popular with actresses including Julia Roberts and singer Geri Halliwell for its ability to transform even the limpest lashes into come-hither fronds. Miniature perming rollers are attached to the lashes with a special glue before a weak perming solution is applied. It's exceptionally effective for short lashes, those with tired eyes or the time-poor, and makes the whole face look fresh and bright. The treatment takes 45 minutes and lasts for approximately three months.

fruit acid peels

All peels use acid to remove layers of skin to reveal the younger, less wrinkled skin beneath, a treatment that is known as skin resurfacing. They range from mild peels, which include the fruit acids, to deep peels which can help sort out damage that lies deeper within the skin. As a rule of thumb, the more intense the peel, the more pain and scabbing you will experience, but the longer-lasting the results will be. I would not recommend much more than a fruit acid peel, which is done in a series of treatments in order to produce results and limit the possibility of scarring.

Derived from sugar cane, glycolic acid (or alphahydroxy acid) in weaker formulations is often mixed into over-the-counter skincare products. 'It's an active ingredient that really works,' says America's leading cosmetic surgeon, Dr Alan Gaynor. 'Glycolic acid makes skin look better by helping aged skin exfoliate more efficiently. It is the increased exfoliation that is responsible for the lovely effects these products can have on your complexion after three months of prolonged use.' A fruit acid peel can help mild acne by opening up blocked pores. There is even some possibility that these products may even reverse some previous sun damage. For moderate-to-deep acne scars, over-the-counter products won't be strong enough. Consult a dermatologist for a fruit acid peel.

laser hair removal

Sometimes called YAG Laser, this is an expensive but safe and gentle non-invasive process that has the same result as electrolysis. This is the hair removal system of the future. Shaving, waxing and hair-removal creams remove unwanted hair, but results are only temporary. The YAG laser is an intense, powerful and focused beam of light which is converted into thermal energy (heat) when it hits a hair containing melanin.

The laser used in cosmetic beauty clinics is strong enough to be effective, but is less powerful than medical lasers which must only be used by doctors because of the risk of burns or de-pigmentation. The YAG laser eliminates unwanted hair without scarring or any side-effects, destroying the hair at the root. It is also practically painless. The ray, which is invisible to the human eye, deeply penetrates the skin, but only the hair stem and follicle absorb the radiation. Unfortunately it cannot be used to remove white hairs, as these contain no melanin and are therefore invisible to the laser. Light hair, fair hair and thin hair contain little melanin, and the treatment might therefore require more sessions. The laser is not suitable for removing unwanted hair that is the result of a hormonal imbalance, rather than a one-off imperfection.

Before treatment with the laser, the skin is cleaned to remove all traces of cosmetics. The hair is then shaved so that all the energy from the laser is directed to the hair bulb, the target of the treatment. After the first session the number of hairs decreases and the remaining hairs begin to thin. Hair goes through three stages of growth, and destruction of the bulb is possible during the active period, so a number of treatments will be needed to eradicate all unwanted hairs completely. Sessions can be repeated every four to five weeks.

This treatment is good for hair you want to remove permanently, such as stray hairs on the chin, rather than eyebrow hairs, but because it leads to redness only use when you have a free day.

I actually couldn't believe this would actually work, but after four sessions my moustache has been almost completely eradicated from my face and doesn't seem to be growing back. I wouldn't consider any more invasive form of cosmetic surgery, but this has been very good value.

Johanna, 31

laser skin resurfacing

One of the most advanced treatments available for reversing the effects of ageing on your skin is the use of short-pulse lasers to vaporize the epidermis. Ageing or damaged skin is delicately removed, layer by layer, with a high-energy beam of light. This is the modern equivalent of a chemical peel, and both treatments expose new skin which is smoother and less wrinkled. Using a laser is cleaner and leads to less pain or swelling, both common side-effects of the chemical approach. Two types of laser are used: carbon dioxide in more severe cases, and an erbium laser which works in a similar way and is good for reversing sun damage, and is also believed to stimulate the production of collagen, which smoothes and firms the skin.

In the case of the CO_2 laser, a powerful beam of carbon dioxide is absorbed by the water in the living cells of your skin. As the water absorbs the energy, the cell and skin are instantly vaporized along with any blood while instantly sealing the nerve endings as layers of skin are gradually removed. 'Magically a lifetime of sun damage, liver spots and pigment irregularity are wiped away,' says leading American cosmetic surgeon Dr Alan Gaynor. Afterwards there is no bleeding, but the skin is raw and a dressing is applied. It takes about two weeks for the red, weepy skin to heal.

My face swelled up and there was a discomfort like a serious sunburn for about a week, but after five days I was back to normal – except I looked at least 10 years younger. Everyone talks about how rested I look and what a glow I have, but they have no idea why.

Shirley, 49

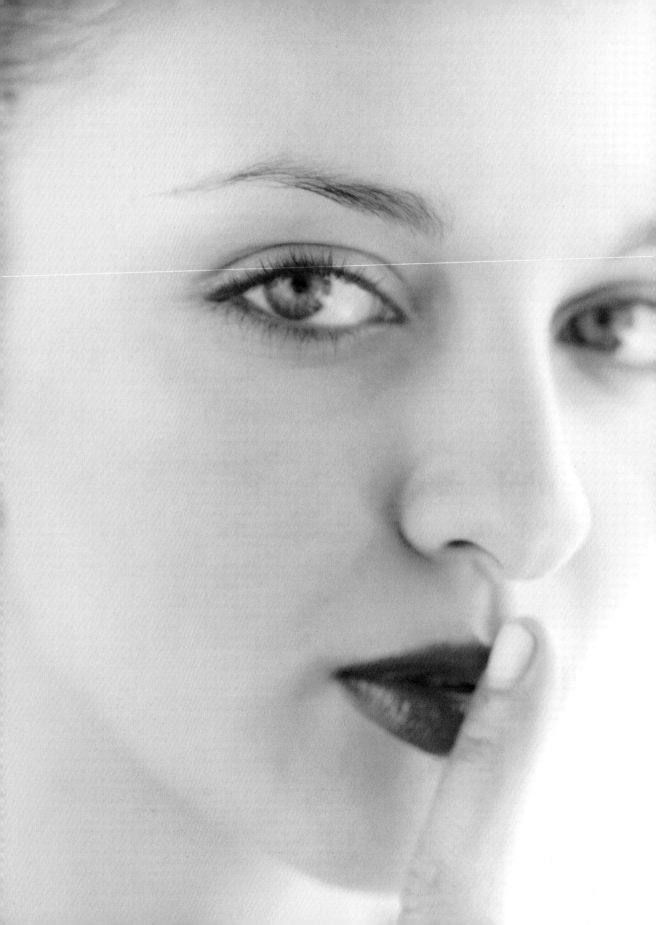

micro-dermabrasion

Micro-dermabrasion is a non-surgical, non-chemical method of skin resurfacing offered at specialist clinics and hospitals. Fine aluminium oxide micro-crystals are expelled through a narrow tube at speed, and this action, together with suction, gently sand-blasts the skin, sloughing away the top dead skin layers. Smoother skin is apparent after just one 30-minute treatment, but it is particularly useful in improving the appearance of acne scars, scar tissue, fine lines and areas of excessive pigmentation. Don't confuse it with dermabrasion, a more invasive treatment using a wheel attached to a rotating device which can go much deeper into the skin and has now largely been replaced by laser treatment, which leads to less swelling and scabbing.

My problem was acne 'cysts' on my cheeks (the sort of red lumps teenage boys tend to get) which didn't show any sign of changing over a period of weeks. The micro-dermabrasion sessions seemed to wear down the lumps bit by bit, with a bit of scabbing at times. It was absolutely brilliant, though, and totally cleared up the problem. Apparently your therapist should keep a watch on how many sessions you have, as it's quite vigorous and your skin can be damaged without due care. Bharti also uses it on stretch marks, and she says the results are really excellent.

Hannah, 54

restylane

This is the brand name given to a synthetic form of hyaloronic acid, a substance that has been used in cataract surgery for over 25 years to keep the eyeball firm during surgery. It is now being used as a wrinkle-filler and as a substitute for collagen injections to lessen the deep lines that can form either side of your nose.

I didn't like the idea of collagen injections, I don't particularly like the idea of acid either, but I had a friend who'd had the treatment and looked years younger while still looking very much like herself. A face-lift has never appealed. This has allowed me to brighten my features, which were getting a bit wrinkled, without looking too obviously 'done'.

Sally, 41

semi-permanent make-up

This is a form of tattooing in which coloured pigments of iron oxide are injected into the skin so that the tiny dots join up and appear to create a band of colour. It is often chosen by women whose eyebrows or eyelashes have thinned, sportswomen or swimmers who do not want to be reapplying make-up constantly, and people who are allergic to make-up or have poor eyesight which makes applying make-up difficult. Some women choose it so they can simply cut out their make-up routine.

Choose a qualified practitioner and ask to see photographic evidence of their work. You need to have faith in their abilities: Any invasive treatment near the eyes carries a risk, and the work they do will be with you for between six months and two years. You should be given an allergy test to ensure you don't react badly to the pigment. Work with the practitioner to create the brow, eye and lip line that feel natural – it can be helpful to draw in your own preference for the practitioner to follow. Colours vary widely, so choose carefully.

An anaesthetic cream is used to numb the area during the treatment, which usually lasts one or two hours. You will be given an antibiotic cream for a week to prevent infection. A top-up session is usually necessary after six weeks or so when the colour will be settled.

As a keen swimmer and athletic coach, I used to have two choices: go out without a streak of make-up, or end up looking a bit of a fright. I didn't have the time or the patience to keep peering into the mirror when training, but I was vain enough to want to look good. I was wary of this tattoo approach to begin with, worried it would look like badly-applied stage make-up, but the results are brilliant, very subtle and incredibly convenient. I've had discrete lip and eye lines drawn on.

Philippa, 38

transdermal electrolysis (TE) system

This non-invasive technique involves the use of an electrical current conducted along the hair shaft into the roots. This is electrolysis without the need for a needle. Current is transmitted from the machine and channelled through tweezers to the unwanted hair. This current chemically changes the water and salt in the follicle to sodium hydroxide. Just as in traditional needle electrolysis, the sodium hydroxide destroys the hair root and papilla, which is the source of nourishment for the hair. The hair doesn't grow back, although you may need a couple of treatments to achieve this, as excessive hair growth can be attributed to many causes, including heredity, stress, hormonal changes and some medications.

No one can predict how many treatments you will need to prevent regrowth, because hair grows in cycles. There can be as many as 1,000 hair follicles or more in a square inch, but less than 100 hairs will be showing at any one time. During the anagen stage, the hair is growing and is visible above the skin, and there is plenty of water and salt in the root area for the current to change chemically. Hair can remain in this stage for two to three weeks.

In the catagen stage, the growth process has stopped, the hair is ready to be shed and the water and salt have dried up, forming a hard bulb. It is not possible to destroy the follicle, and even after treatment another hair will be produced. This stage can last as little as two days.

During the telogen phase, the follicle is dormant and hair is not developing or growing. This phase can last from a few days to a few years, and it is not possible to prevent a hair regrowing when a follicle in this stage is treated with the equipment.

This approach is more painful than waxing, but invaluable for sensitive skin that's prone to scarring.

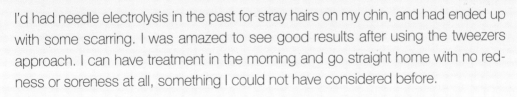

I'd had needle electrolysis in the past for stray hairs on my chin, and had ended up with some scarring. I was amazed to see good results after using the tweezers approach. I can have treatment in the morning and go straight home with no redness or soreness at all, something I could not have considered before.

Jo, 51

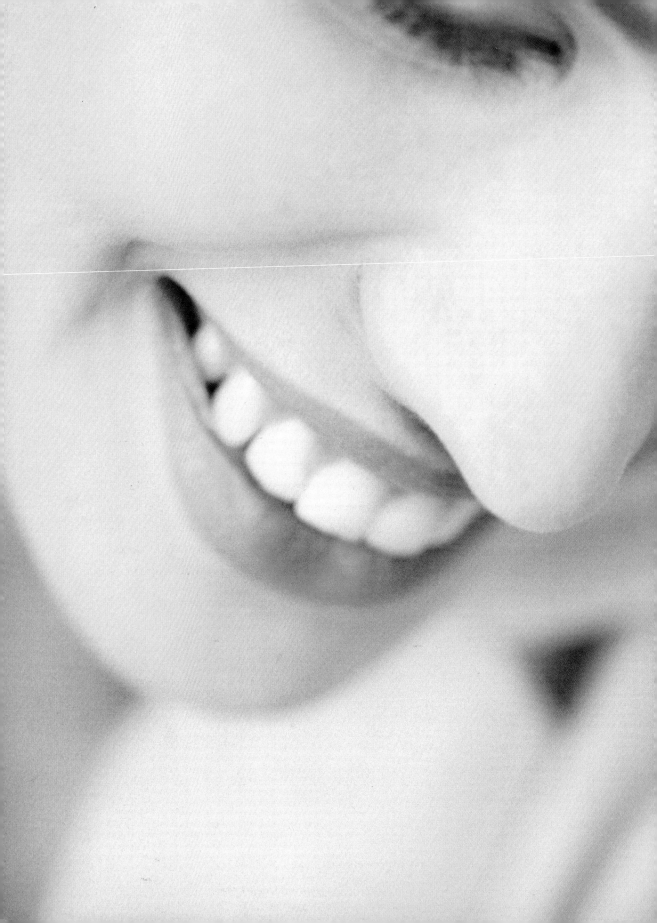

dental treatments

One of the most effective ways to give yourself a lift is cosmetic dentistry. Working on your smile can really improve your confidence. Dr Phil Stemmer, one of the UK's leading aesthetic dentists, is an expert in the art of the Hollywood Smile. Here he gives his insights into the latest treatments, now available in the UK, and what you should expect to pay.

Dr Stemmer's clientele includes actors Jude Law, Sadie Frost, Patsy Kensit and Gary Kemp, and singers from Iron Maiden and Oasis. He offers a range of unique services to confer the confidence-boost given by a youthful, fresh and healthy white smile, and has established Europe's first Fresh Breath Centre using specialist technology to achieve a 95 per cent success rate in cases of bad breath.

Dr Stemmer is the ideal expert to explain processes new to the UK such as 'Power Whitening', a technique that can give a celebrity-white smile in one short visit, and porcelain veneers, which are a big buzz in the US. Scorpio from *Gladiators* asked him to sort out the gap between her two front teeth, of which she had been acutely conscious. After he had applied porcelain veneers to her teeth she was photographed smiling in the newspapers for the first time.

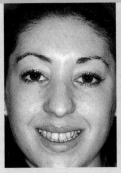
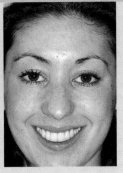
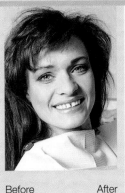
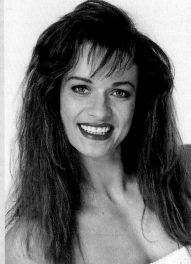

Before   After   Before   After

Power whitening (above, left) can totally change the appearance of a patient's smile.

Porcelain veneers (above, right) can be used to great effect to adjust tooth size and shape.

Gladiator 'Scorpio' (right) is just one of Dr Stemmer's celebrity patients.

The Perfect Smile

We smile most during our fertile years as a means of attracting potential partners. Partly we are showing off our health, as our teeth are at their prime in our youth, but there is other non-verbal communication going on. When men and women are shown photographs of unknown people and asked to rate the perfect smile, for women this is seen as having more rounded teeth with softer edges, while for men squarer teeth are seen as more pleasing. Women smile more in our culture, and often as a signal asking for appeasement, so these softer feminine smiles are a way of seeking approval, whether social or sexual. Mimicking these perfect smiles is usually the goal of the cosmetic dentist.

Celebrity Teeth Costs

Many celebrities are prepared to pay up to £20,000 in search of the perfect smile. Former England star Paul Gascoigne had treatment at Glasgow's HCI Hospital to replace his crooked teeth with a row of shiny new implanted teeth. Actors Tom Cruise, Catherine Zeta Jones and music stars Celine Dion, David Bowie and Ronan Keating have all sought the Hollywood approach. Noel Gallagher spent £10,000 on dental work, Martine McCutcheon invested £15,000 in her smile, and Madonna spent a similar amount giving her teeth a make-over.

how to achieve the hollywood smile

A dazzling, wide, white smile full of perfect teeth is an intensely powerful social weapon, projecting like a laser beam the image of health, vitality and self-assurance. But most of us are not born with teeth like this. Today, the Hollywood smile has become a fashion accessory, created in private cosmetic dental clinics or the sort of one-stop designer smile shops which are becoming a more familiar sight on the high street.

In America, where it all started, politicians and filmstars have discovered that the perfection of a power smile can make the difference between winning and losing a multi-million pound role or earning a place in political office. Everyone from Noel Gallagher to Catherine Zeta Jones, from Donald Trump to Angela Bassett and Stevie Wonder, as well as the cast lists of *Titanic*, *Frasier*, *Seinfeld* and *Friends* have dutifully visited one of the new breed of super-dentists who can give those of us born with dental imperfection – wonky teeth, gap teeth, yellow teeth – the super-smile of our dreams. This is dental work that usually has little to do with filling teeth, gum disease or treating infection, but rather the purposeful creation of a trademark 'power smile'.

Cosmetic dentists work with an artist's eye and a broad palette of new techniques to give the illusion of perfection, deftly manipulating the configuration, colouring and size of teeth. Their expertise is now available in the UK. Forget braces, crowns and bridges. Time-consuming, uncomfortable methods for dental damage have been replaced by rapid, non-surgical procedures which can turn dental defects into something much more appealing. The watchwords here are *porcelain veneers* and *power whitening*.

If you feel your teeth are letting your face down to the extent that you have chosen to invest serious sums in correcting cosmetic problems, read my guide to the latest in aesthetic dentistry, designed to create a smile of Hollywood perfection.

The Britney Spears Smile

The secret here is power whitening.

For decades, Hollywood stars have had their teeth bleached. Recently the young actress Reese Witherspoon had the procedure before the premiere of her film *Legally Blonde* – her cosmetic dental surgeon called it a 'make-or-break smile' – presumably for her, not him!

Just as our hair and skin colour vary, so does teeth colour. Very few people's teeth are actually white – they would look terribly garish if they were. Power-whitening treatment can change the colour of your teeth, brightening your own tooth colour by an average of two to five shades, taking your teeth back to the apparent pearly white-ness of childhood.

Mostly, teeth are shades of ivory or beige. They can become superficially stained with tea, coffee, cola, cranberry juice, tomato juice, smoke, red wine, curry or beetroot juice (stains which can be removed by whitening). But there are four main sources of staining that chemically affect the deeper structure of the tooth and can only be changed by power whitening: ageing, smoking, genetic discolouration and tetracycline stains.

Tetracycline is an antibiotic which, if prescribed before the age of 12, is likely to become incorporated into the structure of growing adult teeth, leading to long-term discoloration which at its worst can make the teeth dark blue, grey or brown. Fortunately, most doctors now know about this side-effect and don't prescribe tetracycline for children. But many older people remain unaware that their teeth have been affected in this way – and that there is a way to solve this aesthetic problem.

Fortunately, modern techniques for whitening the teeth are now more sophisticated than in the past. Hydrogen peroxide has been used for many years to bleach teeth, but it used to have to be heated to the limit of the client's tolerance in order to make an effective chemical reaction. This was quite painful and took several hours. Nowadays we have much quicker treatments using a more sophisticated chemical formula which is chemically more stable and involves no pain (although there can be a bit of sensitivity for a day or two to extremes of hot and cold). There are no other reported side-effects. The whitening process doesn't weaken, damage or make the tooth thinner. Treated teeth are no more susceptible to decay or disease after treatment.

The gums are protected with a rubber guard which also helps keep the lips out of the way, and each tooth is coated with hydrogen peroxide jelly, before being heated with a light for a few minutes to achieve the bleaching process before being washed off with water. At a chemical level the yellow chloride ions in the teeth, which give the tooth its colour, are being swapped with a white ion in the hydrogen peroxide gel. The molecules exchange places – exactly the same process occurs when you dye your hair. At the same time the more superficial food stains are also removed by oxidation.

Results last for approximately six years and the treatment costs from £600, making it the most cost-effective way of making a dramatic change to your smile. Bear in mind that teeth can feel sensitive for the first two days after treatment.

Some British cosmetic dental surgeons follow the treatment up with a Hollywood-style 'take-home tray' – a plastic mould modelled on the client's teeth which is filled with a gentler carbamide peroxide bleaching agent each night and left in while asleep. This is a seven- to ten-day treatment, but take care not to overdo it. You don't want your teeth to look unnaturally white. These are also sold separately from £350 as a budget option.

There are other 'home' kits you can buy over-the-counter to bleach your teeth in the privacy of your own bathroom. They contain a very weak solution, are fairly ineffective and don't give good value for money. A recent article by an American professor who tested these kits found they have a very low pH, which means a very high acidity, leading to potential damage to teeth, fillings and even to crowns.

The other drawback is that, because you don't have a custom-made mouth guard, most of the bleaching chemical leaks out and doesn't stay in contact with the teeth. This can lead to patchy results, as well as pain in the throat and stomach due to swallowing the product. But most importantly, there is no control over colour.

The most dramatic changes are created with the light-activated bleaching agents available only from a dentist, who should carefully protect your gums from temporary discoloration.

The Tom Cruise Smile

The secret here is porcelain veneers.

If you can get away with improving your teeth by using power whitening only, this is by far the best approach and can make a dramatic difference to the way you look. Unfortunately, some people have gaps, decayed teeth, chipped teeth or eroded teeth, and need a bit more help. Porcelain veneers are the answer here. The modern equivalent of caps hide a multitude of sins. A veneer is a thin piece of tooth-coloured porcelain which is attached to the front of the tooth rather in the same way that a false nail is applied to your fingertip, but because teeth don't grow you don't have to have them repaired. On average they are half a millimetre in thickness, just slightly thicker than a nail.

They can be used for straightening teeth or masking discoloured or misaligned teeth, while leaving your own teeth intact underneath. They can make a chipped tooth look perfect again. They also offer a simple way of closing the small gaps between teeth that often make us uncomfortable with our natural smile. Some clients want to use veneers to straighten their teeth; others want their new white veneers made as an exact replica of their own teeth – in either case, the veneers should always look natural.

Because overlays are individually crafted they can be precisely colour-matched, both to other teeth and to the client's skin tone. They can also be made with tiny imperfections to create a lovely, rather than unnaturally perfect, smile. The best are porous and contain oils so the teeth even look constantly glazed and the mouth kissable.

The porcelain used is slightly translucent, just like real teeth, so tiny amounts of light passing through add to the realism. They can also be made to vary in thickness, which enables wonky teeth to be apparently evened out. One of the most effective treatments is having two or four of them fitted over the front teeth, which helps plump out ageing lips – a more effective and safer cosmetic treatment than lip injections.

Earlier caps were often detectable because the metal under-structure was visible at the gum line, but porcelain overlays are applied directly to the tooth enamel, avoiding this. However, they may need to be replaced every 15 to 20 years or so because of wear, chips and any underlying tooth decay. Your teeth also have a natural tendency to deepen in tone as you age, which could make the veneers stand out, but this can be overcome by whitening the teeth in due course if necessary. Unfortunately, veneers can chip like real teeth.

The teeth are prepared by the dentist by filing away some of the natural shiny outer enamel layer of the tooth away to ensure a good bond. Two visits to the cosmetic dentist are usually necessary. At the first visit the tooth is prepared, the shade is matched and a model is taken, which is then sent to a lab where the veneers can be custom-made to fit. On the second visit the veneer is bonded to the tooth with a special adhesive.

Single teeth cost from £600, while an entire power smile could set you back from £4,000–£6,000.

Laser Gum Reshaping

Re-contouring with a laser is used to make the gum look more even. There are many times a patient has one tooth where the gum is too long. The heat of the laser removes the excess gum, automatically cauterizing it. It gives a much more balanced, natural look, and costs from £60 per tooth.

Crowns

Crowns, which are sometimes known as caps, are used to perfect teeth which need to be strengthened, either because they have been broken, have been weakened by a large filling or because of root canal treatment. The crown fits right over the remaining part of the tooth, making it strong and giving it the contour of a natural tooth. New bonding agents and materials such as porcelain and glass make crowns and bridges far less apparent than in the past, but for real strength your best bet is porcelain built up in layers over a precious-metal base. Crowns can look rather obvious if the gums recede with age. A grey line would delineate the edge of the crown, but better-quality ones now come with a porcelain margin, so that even if the gum does recede you won't see the edge. From £500 per tooth.

Bridges and Implants

When you lose a tooth, your appearance isn't the only thing that suffers. The gap left can mean greater strain is applied to the teeth either side, and they can end up leaning into the gap, which can affect your 'bite' (the way your teeth lock together when you chew). There are three main ways to replace the missing teeth. The first is a partial denture, using a removable false tooth or teeth. The second is with a bridge, which is often used when there are fewer teeth to replace. This is made by constructing crowns on the teeth either side of the gap and joining them together with a false tooth in the middle. The whole lot is cemented into place with special glue. The third process is an implant: a metal root is painlessly placed into the bone and a crown or cap is fitted onto it. These are hassle-free methods of replacement, but their realism goes further: You have to clean them every day. From £1,000.

Sealants

These are effective thin plastic coatings, applied as a liquid which then hardens like a varnish, which can be applied to children's teeth to seal crevices in the rear molars from the age of six. These act as a barrier to prevent bacteria collecting deep down within the fine fissures of the tooth beyond the reach of a toothbrush, which leads to decay. It's a painless treatment, popular with switched-on British parents, that changes the crevices in their children's teeth from a V-shape into a U-shape, making cleaning easier. It doesn't affect the 'bite' of the teeth (the way the upper and lower jaws lock together), because the sealant fills only the fine contours of the tooth. From £25 per tooth.

White Fillings

Private dentists can now replace dull grey amalgam fillings with semi-translucent fillings made from porcelain, or a hybrid of quartz or glass, which is perfectly matched to the colour tone of the surrounding tooth. They take longer to set and are more expensive than amalgam, but they are safer and look nicer. From £80 a tooth.

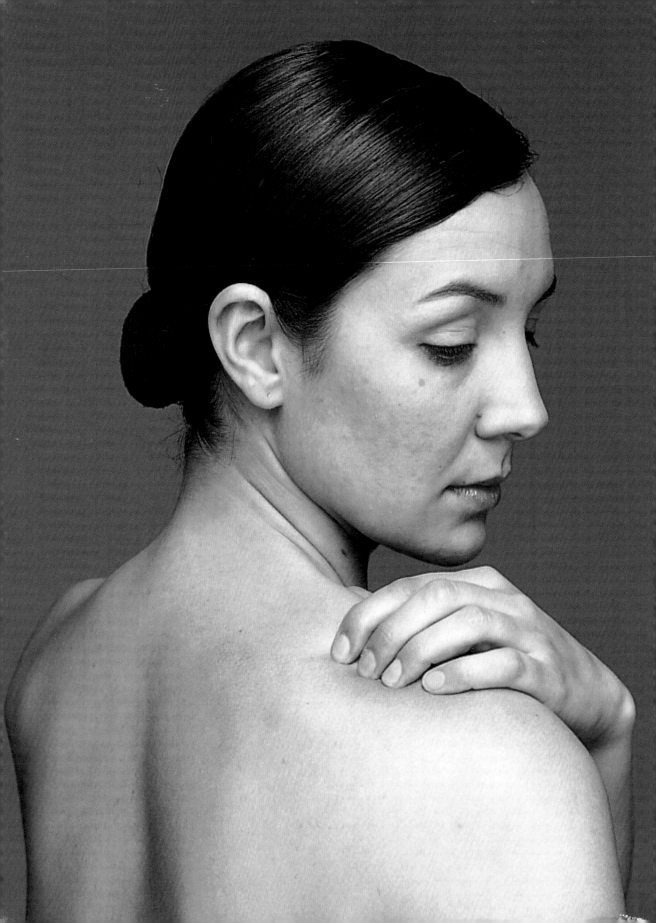

resources

Bharti Vyas

Bharti Vyas clinic and skincare range is available from Selfridges, larger House of Fraser stores and selected clinics. Bharti also produces an affordable skincare range for Tesco – Skin Wisdom.

The Bharti Vyas Training Centre

Bharti Vyas holds regular seminars at her Training Centre in central London. These one day seminars are specifically designed to give the individual the knowledge and power to take control of his or her own well-being and to make the BV philosophy a way of life. The seminars are also open to couples who want to help each other look after themselves, reduce stress and enjoy energy and vitality. Each individual is furnished with notes from the seminar.

For further information, please visit the website at: www.bharti-vyas.co.uk or telephone: 020 7486 7910

Bharti Vyas
Training Centre
57 George Street
London WIU 8LX

Dental Care

www.dentistry.com
For up-to-date articles on the latest American treatments, such as power whitening, porcelain veneers, etc.

Dr Phil Stemmer

Teeth for Life Clinic
Conan Doyle House
2 Devonshire Place
London W1G 6HJ
020 7935 7511/020 7935 0407

Tongue Care

Dental Health Boutique

0800 454 806

For professionally-designed tongue-scrapers

Fresh Breath

Fresh Breath Centre

www.freshbreath.co.uk
email: fresh.breath@virgin.net
020 7935 7511
The Fresh Breath Centre was founded in 1995 by Dr Phil Stemmer B.D.S and Prof. Mel Rosenburg, oral microbiologist and leading authority on breath odour. There are two centres in the UK.

Eco-conscious Skincare Products

Aveda

www.aveda.com

020 7410 1600 for stockists

Aveda products are made from pure plant and flower derivatives and are entirely free from petrochemicals.

Essential Oils

Findhorn Flower Essences

www.findhornessences.com

email: info@findhornessences.com

Flower Essence Repertoire

www.ifer.co.uk

email: flowers@atlas.co.uk

Eyebrows

www.eyebrowz.com

This website was set up by Nancy Parker, the American eyebrow guru, and is packed full of step-by-step information for creating the perfect brow, eyebrow make-overs, and products for sale such as eyebrow stencils inspired by celebrity shapes as well as those based on the five basic eyebrow shapes.

Glasses

www.luxotticagroup.com

This website that provides an in-depth guide to choosing the right frame shape for your face shape. Click on 'Selecting eye wear' and then on 'Face shape guide'.

Natural Health

www.revital.com

For a wide range of organic foods, natural supplements, herbal remedies, natural skin-care products, aloe vera and flower essences

www.nutricentre.co.uk

For a wide range of supplements, herbs, tinctures, flower remedies and other natural products

Skin Conditions

www.yourskin.co.uk

www.talkeczema.com

For advice on skin disorders, including eczema

Jackson Ltd

01923 853111

www.taylor-jackson.com

For cream, bath oil or herbal extract with *Mahonia aquifolium*, which can help to ease eczema symptoms

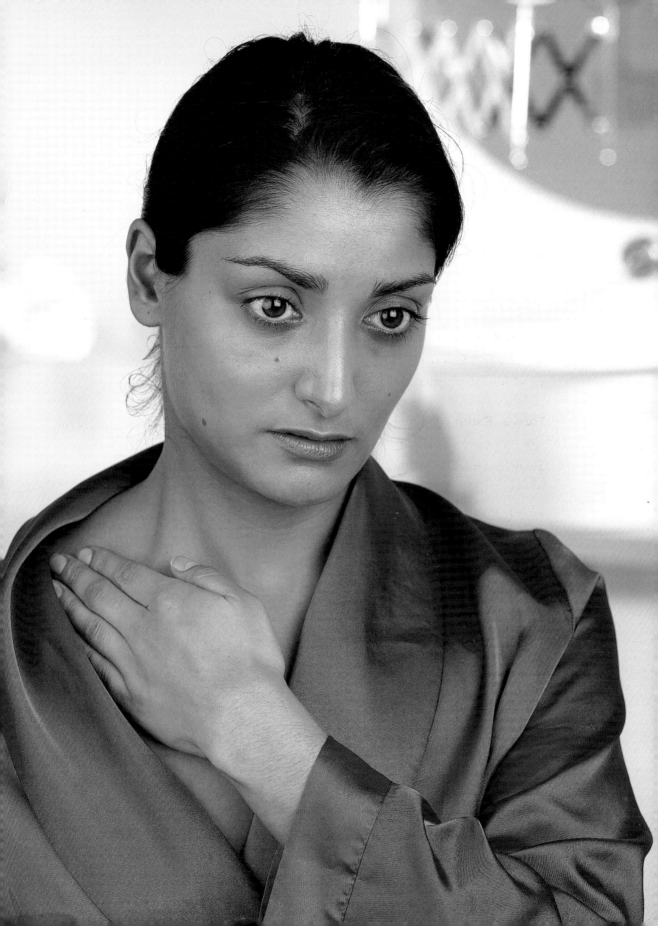

further reading

Acupressure for Health, Jacqueline Young (Thorsons)

Acupressure Made Easy, Dr Julian Kenyon (Thorsons)

The Art of Indian Face Massage, Narendra Mehta (Thorsons)

Beautiful Brows, Nancy Parker (Three Rivers Press)

The Beauty Bible, Sarah Stacey and Josephine Fairley (Kyle Cathie)

Complete Family Guide to Dental Health, Barrie Sherman and Anne Sherman (Thorsons)

Cosmetics Unmasked, Dr Stephen & Gina Antczak (Thorsons)

Get Well, Stay Well, Dr Paul Sherwood with Claire Haggard (Thorsons)

Give Your Face A Lift: Natural Ways to Look Good, Penny Stanway (Ulysses Press)

The Good Skin Doctor, Dr Anthony C. Chu & Anne Lovell (Thorsons)

How to Wash Your Face, Barney J. Kenet, M.D with Patricia Lawler (Simon & Schuster)

Indian Head Massage, Narendra Mehta (Thorsons First Directions)

The Lowdown on Facelifts and Other Wrinkle Remedies, Wendy Lewis (Quadrille)

Natural Recipes for Perfect Skin, Pierre Jean Cousin (Quadrille)

Perfect Skin: The Natural Approach, Amanda Cochrane (Piatkus)

Skin Tricks: Tools of the Trade, Dr Gerald Imber (Thorsons)

Stop Ageing Now, Jean Carper (Thorsons)

Super Skin, Kathryn Marsden (Thorsons)

Timeless Face: 30 days to a Younger You, Ellae Elinwood (St Martin's Griffin)

Bharti Vyas is also the author of these bestselling guides:

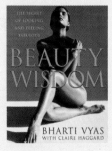

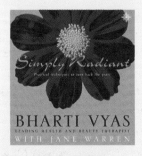

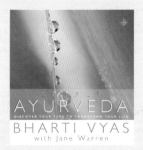

Beauty Wisdom　　　　*Simply Radiant*　　　　*Simply Ayurveda*

skin wisdom

Created for Tesco by Bharti Vyas

Skin Wisdom is a comprehensive range of quality skincare products that have been developed to work in harmony to restore your skin to its optimum condition and protect it from the outside elements. I live by a simple philosophy that beauty on the outside begins on the inside and have reflected this in the creation of the Skin Wisdom range.

I am delighted to have teamed up with Tesco to create the first supermarket skincare range developed by a professional holistic beauty therapist. This unique partnership has enabled us to offer salon quality, superior skincare to everyone at affordable prices. By using a Skin Wisdom product you will become your own therapist, reaping all the benefits of professional beauty treatments in your own home.

Skin Wisdom Range

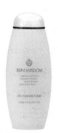
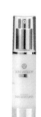

Cleanser
Facial Wash Gel
Alcohol Free Toner
2-In-1 Cleanser Toner
Eye Make-Up Remover
12 Hour Daily Moisturiser
SPF 6 Daily Moisturiser
Intensive Night Cream
3-In-1 Cleansing Wipes For Dry
   & Sensitive Skin
Oil Balancing 3-In-1 Cleansing Wipes
Age Defying 3-In-1 Cleansing Wipes
Cleansing Mask
Thermal Clay Mask
Vitamin Recovery F.A.C.E. Mask
2-In-1 Facial Scrub & Mask
Gentle Facial Scrub
Refreshing Eye Pads
Body Lotion
Softening Salt Butter Rub
Hip & Thigh Toning Gel

Cooling Body Slush
Hydrating Body Wash
Crème Bath
Sheer Radiance Body Moisturiser

Skin Wisdom Extra Care Range

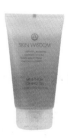
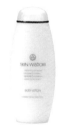
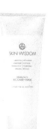
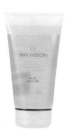

Age Defying Daily Moisturiser
Age Defying Night Firming Cream
Age Defying Eye Cream
Age Defying Radiance Serum
Age Defying Body Cream
Age Defying Hand & Nail Cream
Pre Sun Tan Accelerator For Face
Anti-Ageing Sun Protection For Face
   SPF 25
Self Tan Mousse For Face & Body
Soothing Aftersun Recovery Mask For Face
Firming Aftersun Moisturiser
Tan Maximising Aftersun

index

acne 27–31, 129, 155
acupressure 101–2, 109–12
age spots 34–5, 128
ageing 19–25, 47, 113, 134, 141–2, 161
alpha hydroxy acid 17

bad breath 74–6, 175
birthmarks 129
blackheads 32–3, 155
blemishes 27–36, 129
blusher 152
botox 157
bridges 173

chemicals 55–6, 153–5
cleansing 9–12, 42, 44
collagen 3, 23–4, 157
combination skin 7–8, 149
conditioners 62, 65
crowns 172
crow's feet 81
curly hair 55

dandruff 56, 65
dark circles 80–1
dentistry 69, 167–73, 175
dermis 3, 37
dry hair 53–4
dry skin 6–7, 12, 16–17, 37, 43, 148
dull skin 142, 149

eczema 33–4, 155, 176
elastin 4
electrolysis 165
epidermis 3
exercises 93, 113–23
eyes 77–91
    ageing 142
    bags 32, 80–1
    brows 84–7, 141, 176
    care 82
    colour 138
    lashes 83, 159
    massage 78
    treatments 47

face
    exercises 113–23
    hair 26–7, 160
    masks 25, 44–5
    massage 93–123
    shapes 50–2, 85–90, 130–5
    toning 117–23
fillings 173
flaky skin 17
flossing 69, 71
foundation 149–50
freckles 128–9
fruit acid peels 159

glasses 129–30, 176
greasy hair 54–5
greying hair 57
gums 70–1

hair 49–67
head massage 94–100
home-made treatments 41–7, 61–7

implants 173

jargon 143–4

laser treatments 160–1, 172
lice 56–7
lymph 103–4

make-up 12, 126–55, 164
makeovers 137–40
massage techniques 95–100
mayo-lift 158
micro-dermabrasion 162
moisturizers 15–17, 43
moles 35
mouthwash 69, 73–4, 76

natural make-up 146–7
normal skin 5, 8, 12, 17

oily skin 6–8, 12, 16, 42, 148
open pores 148

permed hair 55–6
polishing 13–14, 24, 43–4
professional insights 144–5
psoriasis 35–6
puffy eyes 81–2

red eyes 80
restylane 163
rosacea 30–1

scalp massage 66, 94–5
sealants 173
shampoo 62
shaving 90
shiny hair 67
sight problems 129–30
skin 5–8, 148–9
    ageing 141–2
    care 175–6
    colour 135
    disorders 27–36
    feeding 18
    layers 2–4
    resurfacing 159, 161
    tags 36
soap 10, 46
spectacles 129–30, 176
spots 27–9, 129
Stemmer, P. 69, 72–6, 167, **175**
stretching exercises 114–16
subcutis 4
sunscreen 38–9
sunshine 37–9

T-zone 7, 149
tea tree oil 31
teeth 69–76, 167–73
thinning hair 58
threading 90
thyroid 19, 81
tired eyes 78
tongue 72, 175
toning 14
toothpaste 73
tweezing 90–1

warts 36
wrinkles 24–5